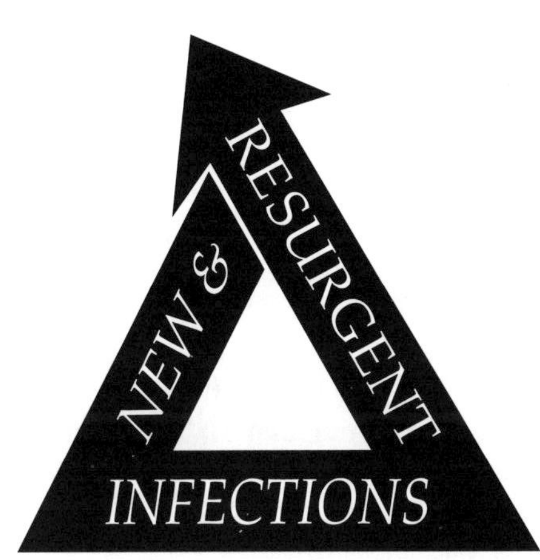
NEW &
RESURGENT
INFECTIONS

Also available in the Wiley Series of *London School of Hygiene & Tropical Medicine* Annual Public Health Forums...

DIET, NUTRITION & CHRONIC DISEASE
Lessons from Contrasting Worlds
Edited by PRAKASH S. SHETTY and KLIM McPHERSON
0471 97133 2 301pp 1997
Sixth Annual Public Health Forum

HEALTH AT THE CROSSROADS
Transport Policy and Urban Health
Edited by TONY FLETCHER and ANTHONY J. McMICHAEL
0471 96272 4 354pp 1996
Fifth Annual Public Health Forum

VACCINATION AND WORLD HEALTH
Edited by F.T. CUTTS and P.G. SMITH
0471 95242 7 308pp 1995
Fourth Annual Public Health Forum

TUBERCULOSIS
Back to the Future
Edited by JOHN PORTER and KEITH McADAM
0471 94346 0 304pp (pr) 1993
Third Annual Public Health Forum

EUROPE WITHOUT FRONTIERS
The Implications for Health
Edited by CHARLES E.M. NORMAND and PATRICK VAUGHAN
0471 93761 4 396pp (pr) 1993
0471 93759 2 396pp (cl) 1993
Second Annual Public Health Forum

MALARIA
Waiting for the Vaccine
Edited by GEOFFREY TARGETT
0471 93100 4 236pp 1991
First Annual Public Health Forum

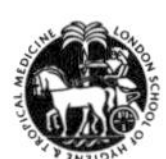

London School of Hygiene & Tropical Medicine
Seventh Annual Public Health Forum

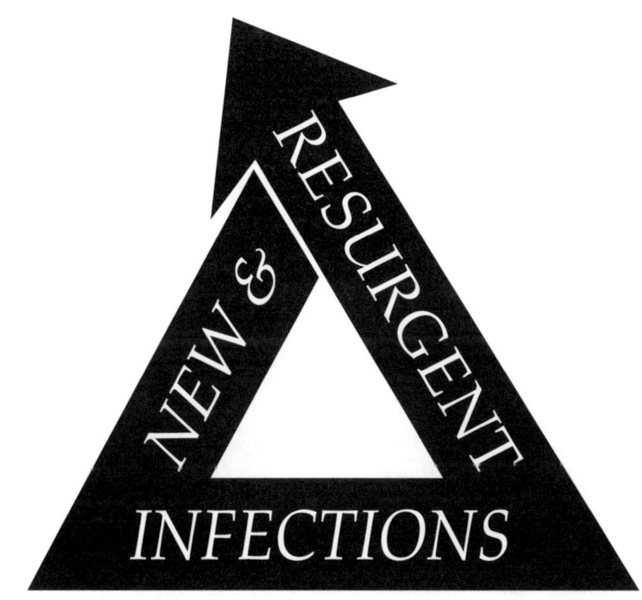

Prediction, Detection and Management of Tomorrow's Epidemics

Edited by
Brian Greenwood and Kevin De Cock

Series Editor
Alice Dickens

London School of Hygiene & Tropical Medicine, London, UK

JOHN WILEY & SONS

Chichester · New York · Weinheim · Brisbane · Singapore · Toronto

National 01243 779777
International (+44) 1243 779777
e-mail (for orders and customer service enquiries): cs-books@wiley.co.uk
Visit our Home Page on http://www.wiley.co.uk or http://www.wiley.com

Other Wiley Editorial Offices

John Wiley & Sons, Inc., 605 Third Avenue,
New York, NY 10158-0012, USA

WILEY-VCH Verlag GmbH, Pappelallee 3,
D-69469 Weinheim, Germany

Jacaranda Wiley Ltd, 33 Park Road, Milton,
Queensland 4064, Australia

John Wiley & Sons (Asia) Pte Ltd, 2 Clementi Loop #02-01,
Jin Xing Distripark, Singapore 129809

John Wiley & Sons (Canada) Ltd, 22 Worcester Road,
Rexdale, Ontario M9W 1LI, Canada

Library of Congress Cataloging-in-Publication Data

London School of Hygiene & Tropical Medicine Public Health Forum (7th : 1998)
New and resurgent infections : prediction, detection, and management of tomorrow's epidemics / London School of Hygiene & Tropical Medicine Seventh Annual Public Health Forum: edited by Brian Greenwood and Kevin De Cock.
p. cm.
Includes bibliographical references and index.
ISBN 0-471-98174-5 (hardcover)
1. Epidemiology—Congresses. 2. Communicable disease—Congresses. I. Greenwood, B. M. II. De Cock, Kevin. III. Title.
[DNLM: 1. Communicable Diseases—epidemiology—congresses.
2. Communicable Disease Control—congresses. 3. Drug Resistance—congresses. WC 100 L847n 1988]
RA651.L66 1988
614.4—dc21 97–46506
CIP

British Library Cataloguing in Publication Data

A catalogue record for this book is available from the British Library

ISBN 0-471-98174-5

Typeset in 10/12pt Times from the author's disks by Vision Typesetting, Manchester
Printed and bound in Great Britain by Biddles Ltd, Guildford and King's Lynn
This book is printed on acid-free paper responsibly manufactured from sustainable forestry, in which at least two trees are planted for each one used for paper production.

Contents

Contributors

Ruth L. Berkelman, National Center for Infectious Diseases, Centers for Disease Control and Prevention, Atlanta, GA, USA

David J. Bradley, Department of Infectious and Tropical Diseases, London School of Hygiene & Tropical Medicine, Keppel Street, London WC1E 7HT, UK

Jean Buzby, Economic Research Service, US Department of Agriculture, Washington DC, USA

Kevin M. De Cock, Department of Infectious and Tropical Diseases, London School of Hygiene & Tropical Medicine, Keppel Street, London WC1E 7HT, UK

Paul R. Epstein, Center for Health and the Global Environment, Harvard Medical School, Boston, USA

Susan Foster, Department of Public Health & Policy, London School of Hygiene & Tropical Medicine, Keppel Street, London WC1E 7HT, UK

Melba Gomes, Special Programme for Research and Training in Tropical Diseases, World Health Organization, CH-1211 Geneva 27, Switzerland

Brian A. Greenwood, Department of Infectious and Tropical Diseases, London School of Hygiene & Tropical Medicine, Keppel Street, London WC1E 7HT, UK

Duane J. Gubler, Division of Vector-Borne Infectious Diseases, National Center for Infectious Diseases, Centers for Disease Control and Prevention, US Department of Health and Human Services, PO Box 2087, Fort Collins, CO 80522, USA

Mitiku Haile, Mekelle University College, Mekelle, Ethiopia

David L Heymann, Division of Emerging and Other Communicable Diseases Surveillance and Control, World Health Organization, 1211 Geneva 27, Switzerland

T. Jacob John, Christian Medical College and Hospital, PO Box 3, Vellore 632 004, India

Luc Kestens, Laboratory of Immunology, Institute of Tropical Medicine, Nationalestraat 155, B-2000 Antwerpen, Belgium

Thomas G. Ksiazek, Special Pathogens Branch, National Center for Infectious Diseases, Centers for Disease Control and Prevention, Atlanta, GA, USA

Bruce R. Levin, Department of Biology, Emory University, Atlanta, GA, USA

Jordan Lin, Economic Research Service, US Department of Agriculture, Washington, DC, USA

Kenneth Linthicum, Department of Epidemiology, Armed Forces Research Institute for Medicine, Bangkok, Thailand

Lindsay J. Martinez, Division of Emerging and Other Communicable Diseases Surveillance and Control, World Health Organization, 1211 Geneva 27, Switzerland

Andrew McMichael, Institute of Molecular Medicine, John Radcliffe Hospital, Oxford, UK

Anthony J. McMichael, Department of Epidemiology and Population Health, London School of Hygiene & Tropical Medicine, Keppel Street, London WC1E 7HT, UK

Paul Mead, Centers for Disease Control and Prevention, Atlanta, GA, USA

Alain Moren, European Programme for Intervention Epidemiology Training, Reseau National de Santé Publique, Paris, France

Gilbert Mpigika, Malaria Control Unit, Ministry of Health, PO Box 8, Entebbe, Uganda

Peggy Nunnery, The Food Safety and Inspection Service, US Department of Agriculture, Washington, DC, USA

Stephen R. Palmer, Welsh Combined Centres for Public Health, University of Wales College of Medicine, Abton House, Wedal Road, Cardiff CF4 3QX, Wales

Tanya Roberts, Economic Research Service, US Department of Agriculture, Washington, DC, USA

Pierre E. Rollin, Special Pathogens Branch, National Center for Infectious Diseases, Centers for Disease Control and Prevention, Atlanta, GA, USA

Anthony Sanchez, Special Pathogens Branch, National Center for Infectious Diseases, Centers for Disease Control and Prevention, Atlanta, GA, USA

Peter G. Smith, Department of Infectious and Tropical Diseases, London School of Hygiene & Tropical Medicine, Keppel Street, London WC1E 7HT, UK

Phillip I. Tarr, University of Washington School of Medicine, Seattle, WA, USA

Guido Vanham, Laboratory of Immunology, Institute of Tropical Medicine, Nationalestraat 155, B-2000 Antwerpen, Belgium

Sherif R. Zaki, Infectious Disease Pathology Activity, National Center for Infectious Diseases, Centers for Disease Control and Prevention, Atlanta, GA, USA

Foreword

David Nabarro

UK Department for International Development (formerly the UK Overseas Development Administration)

I was delighted that DFID was able to sponsor the London School of Hygiene & Tropical Medicine's Seventh Annual Public Health Forum. This was an important meeting, examining a topical and serious public health issue—new and resurgent infections.

When I trained in public health at the London School of Hygiene & Tropical Medicine in 1979, the general view was that the suffering caused throughout the world by infectious diseases would fall because of the availability of improved preventive measures. Yet evidence from recent studies of the global burden of disease reminds us that infectious diseases continue to cause enormous hardship, particularly in the poorest communities of the world. Some of these diseases have been with us for many decades, refusing to be tamed despite efforts to develop and implement preventive measures. Others have come back, displaying new-found resistance to antibiotics and control measures.

Those who invest their precious time and energy in research in the life sciences accept that from time to time their propositions turn out to be wrong. This does not mean they have failed: the disproving of hypotheses is an important contributor to the development of our collective knowledge and our understanding of what is happening in the world.

But those of us working in public health, who give advice to those allocating resources, have to accept that the consequences of being wrong are sometimes costly. We have to give our advice in a way which takes account of uncertainty. We seek knowledge that is synthesized in a way that takes account of risks and assumptions. We push scientists to give us predictions with ever-narrowing confidence intervals. The better the predictions, the more useful the advice we can offer.

Spare a thought, though, for those on the receiving end of our uncertainty. There are the legislators, who have to make difficult choices about the allocation of scarce resources. They depend on our advice while doing this, and have to take responsibility for the consequences of their decisions. They may not always be able to allocate resources in a way which reflects the greatest margin of safety for people's health. They have to operate within a context of, and often choose between, competing demands. This book seeks to identify the individual, professional and institutional responses that are most likely to be effective in reducing threats to public health from new and resurgent infections.

We are pleased that the World Health Organization has increased its attention to infectious diseases, and has become involved in both examining and advising on new and resurgent infections through its division of emerging and other communicable disease surveillance and control. The World Health Organization has a legitimate right to act, on behalf of its new member states, in establishing a coherent global response to new and resurgent infections. This work will be particularly relevant to the poorest 25% of the world's population, who suffer excessively, and die young, as a result of infectious diseases.

On behalf of the UK Government's Department for International Development, I welcome this important publication. The guidance that it offers to the scientific community, public health professionals, legislators, and the different parts of the World Health Organization and other UN systems agencies will help those who are most affected by new and resurgent infections, both now and in the future.

Preface

Kevin De Cock

The 20th century opened with infectious diseases dominating medicine and witnessed scientific advances that promised control over them; it closes with abundant reminders that the history of infectious disease is unfinished. The renewed interest in infection in the 1990s led the London School of Hygiene & Tropical Medicine to devote its 1997 Annual Public Health Forum to the subject of new and resurgent infections.

Edward Jenner conducted his experiments on vaccination against smallpox in England in the late 18th century, when physicians had little scientific understanding of disease pathogenesis. The 19th century saw great advances in microbiology, epidemiology and public health, with the work, among others, of John Snow on cholera, Robert Koch on tuberculosis, and Louis Pasteur on rabies and other infections. The 19th century in Europe produced infrastructure for sanitation, waste disposal, and safe water supplies, established the disciplines of bacteriology and parasitology, and created institutes such as the London School devoted to public health and tropical medicine. These scientific advances were in turn applied to improving health overseas in the colonies of the European empires.

Progress in medicine over the present century has been extraordinary. The development of safe anaesthesia, blood transfusion and intensive care has greatly reduced the dangers of surgery and obstetrics. Certain cancers have become curable, organ transplantation has become routine, and molecular biology and genetics hold promise for the future. Most spectacularly, the development of effective antimicrobial drugs and of a wide variety of vaccines has led to the cure and prevention of many infectious diseases, and to the eradication of one ancient scourge, smallpox. It is understandable, therefore, that students training in medicine in the second half of this century concluded that infectious diseases were a receding threat, and that research and public health should focus on other priorities.

Today, this optimism seems premature. Infectious diseases have always been the leading cause of death in developing countries, but account for a substantial and sometimes increasing burden of disease in industrialized nations. An impressive number of new infectious agents have recently been discovered, some with consequences no one could have foreseen. HIV/AIDS must be considered the 'mother of all emerging infections' which, within 10 years of its recognition, had become the leading cause of death in young adult men in the USA, had begun to erase hard-won gains in child survival in many African cities, and had been responsible for a doubling or tripling of tuberculosis cases in some countries. Outbreaks of other new infections have also occurred, sometimes with very high mortality, as exemplified by the haemorrhagic fevers due to Ebola, Lassa and Marburg viruses.

Apart from new diseases, we have also witnessed a resurgence of some infections which were previously well controlled. The USA first documented the resurgence of tuberculosis in 1985 and this has been seen subsequently in some other industrialized countries. The former Soviet Union has suffered a severe epidemic of diphtheria which is only now coming under control, as well as a severe resurgence of syphilis. An important but neglected epidemic of human African trypanosomiasis is currently under way in the former Zaire. Urban yellow fever occurred in Western Nigeria in 1986 for the first time anywhere in the world for 40 years, and yellow fever has also occurred recently in Kenya, having been absent from East Africa for decades. In 1994, the world's attention was drawn to an outbreak of plague in Surat, India, an outbreak with many lessons about the international response to epidemics, and which had huge financial and social consequences.

Finally, we have also experienced the development and spread of resistance to the drugs available to combat infectious diseases. Multi-drug resistant tuberculosis (MDRTB) came to attention in New York City, where institutional outbreaks occurred in the early 1990s with high mortality, mostly involving HIV-infected persons. The spread of this problem to developing countries with high rates of HIV infection, should it occur, has the potential to render tuberculosis once more an incurable disease. When half a million or more refugees streamed into Zaire from Rwanda following the genocidal events of mid-1994, epidemic cholera as well as shigellosis occurred, shigellosis that was resistant to all drugs except ciprofloxacin. If quinolone resistance develops, East and Central Africa will face *Shigella* infection for which we have no effective antimicrobial therapy. Other diseases affected by drug resistance with public health implications include chloroquine-resistant malaria and penicillin-resistant gonorrhoea and pneumococcal infection. In industrialized countries, hospital wards are sometimes closed for control of methicillin-resistant *Staphylococcus aureus*.

Concern about national preparedness to address infectious diseases has led the Institute of Medicine of the US National Academy of Sciences to issue several reports since the late 1980s. Its third report, entitled *Emerging infections: microbial threats to health in the United States* (1992), has been seminal in defining the concept of emerging and re-emerging infectious diseases, and laying the basis for a response. The Centers for Disease Control and Prevention published a plan in 1994 (CDC, 1994) addressing the priorities outlined by the Insitute of Medicine and defining the necessary response to emerging infectious diseases.

To underline the seriousness with which this topic is taken, an interagency working group was set up by the US Government in 1994 to examine the global threat posed by emerging infections. The working group was chaired by Dr

David Satcher, CDC's Director, and included representatives from more than 17 different US Government agencies, including its most prominent, such as the Departments of State, Defence, and Agriculture, as well as the National Institutes of Health. Vice President Gore has shown particular interest in the work of this group. Recent events in the UK concerning food safety, such as the outbreaks of bovine spongiform encephalitis (BSE), new variant Creutzfeldt–Jakob disease and *E.coli* 0157:*H*7 illustrate how emerging infections can quickly become relevant to the highest levels of government.

Against this background, the suggestion was made last year by Professor Michael Miles, supported by Professor Geoffrey Targett, both of the Department of Medical Parasitology at the School, that the 1997 Annual Public Health Forum should be devoted to the subject of new and resurgent infections. Professor Brian Greenwood and I were invited to be the Chair and Director of the Conference, respectively, with the organization capably managed by Alice Dickens. Staff across the School contributed to the development of the programme. The aims of the Forum were to review the subject of emerging infections, to assess our preparedness for addressing emerging infections, to consider future prospects and to define the appropriate public health response and research.

To our knowledge, this conference represented the first large-scale meeting on emerging infections to be held in Europe. A noteworthy feature distinguishing it from the numerous meetings held in North America on this topic was the participation of many delegates from the developing world, where infectious disease epidemiology is also changing, although less closely observed. Discussants were asked to question the originality of the concept of infectious disease emergence in socio-economic environments where microbial threats have always dominated medicine. The international nature of the conference was one of its most rewarding and stimulating aspects, and we hope this is conveyed in these published proceedings. The School is most grateful to the following organizations, who generously sponsored the Forum, and without whose contributions the Forum would not have been possible: the UK Department for International Development (formerly the Overseas Development Administration), US Centers for Disease Control and Prevention, US National Institutes of Health and the Fogarty International Center, the Wellcome Trust, the World Health Organization, and Glaxo Wellcome who sponsored the publication of this book.

Momentous changes have occurred over the 20th century, now in its final years: whole empires have been dismantled, world wars have been fought, extraordinary biomedical advances have occurred. The pace of social and biological change in the 21st century will continue to increase, with as yet uncertain consequences for infectious agents or human interactions with them. The essential lesson from the now dying 20th century is that infectious agents share the ecosystem with us; while we may control many infectious diseases through judicious medical and public health practice, vigilance can never be relaxed.

References

Centers for Disease Control. *Addressing emerging infectious disease threats: a prevention strategy for the United States.* Atlanta, GA: Centers for Disease Control and Prevention, Public Health Service, US Department of Health and Human Services, 1994

Institute of Medicine. *Emerging infections: microbial threats to health in the United States.* Washington, DC: National Academy Press, 1992

1
The influence of local changes in the rise of infectious disease

David J. Bradley

London School of Hygiene & Tropical Medicine, UK

This chapter tackles the question of how diseases emerge. The processes that lead to the emergence of infections are diverse and many-layered. Some are quite local and specific but may have great consequences—along the lines of the story of a battle lost for want of a horseshoe nail—while others are on a much greater scale, such as global warming. The dominant answer to this question for much of this century has been a meso-scale answer or microbiological explanation. When a pathogen has been identified we feel we understand the disease that has emerged. Identification of an outbreak as one of yellow fever sums up the whole natural history of the outbreak: its aetiology, transmission, pathogenesis and public health implications. However, attaching a microbiological label to an outbreak is not a complete answer, for it does not answer either the micro-scale questions such as 'why is there an outbreak here, now, of this size, affecting these people?', nor does it answer the macro-questions such as 'why are there more (or fewer) outbreaks this decade than last?' Nor does it answer the question 'what drives the overall worldwide trends in such problems?'

This chapter attempts to address these questions about 'why'. There is a continuous spectrum of answers from the ultra-micro to the global. The chapter by Anthony McMichael (this volume, chapter 2) looks at the grand scale while the present chapter focuses on the micro-scale. It is clear that these approaches are sometimes simply different ways of looking at the same question: the global problem of misuse of medicines leading to emergence of drug-resistant microorganisms is Mr Bukanga taking inadequate doses of an inappropriate antibiotic multiplied a hundred thousand times. Yet there are uses to this division. Macro problems require macro solutions. Global warming cannot be stopped by small-scale individual action but raises problems of political will and

New and Resurgent Infections: Prediction, Detection and Management of Tomorrow's Epidemics.
Edited by B. Greenwood and K. De Cock.

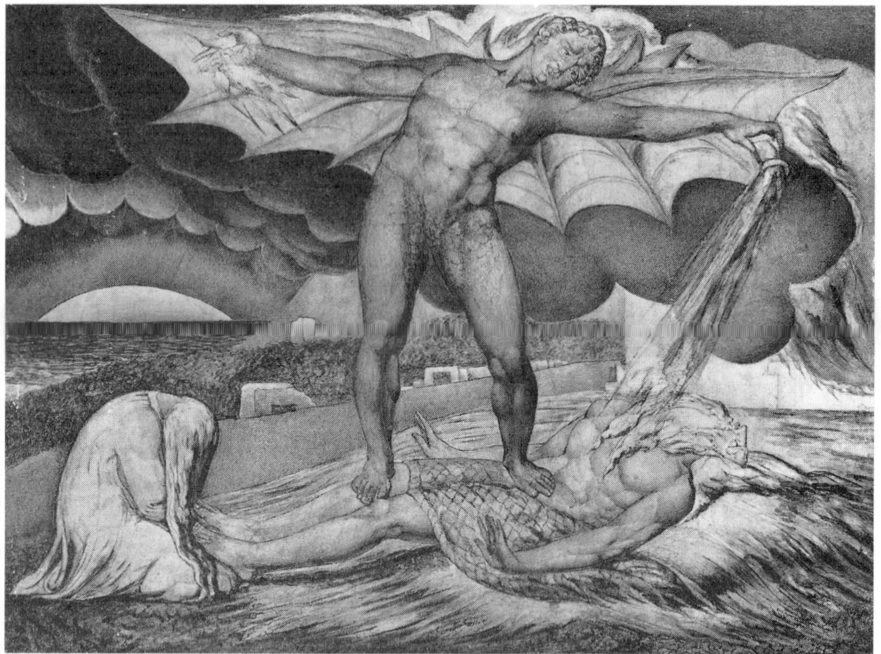

Figure 1.1 William Blake: *Satan smiting Job with sore boils*. Reproduced with the permission of the Trustees of the Tate Gallery, London

national policy. Prevention of emerging diseases depends on the appropriate mixture of large- and small-scale interventions with changes in environment and in human behaviour.

Micro-level considerations address some of the questions raised by the worried public health official today, and before that by the shaman, witch doctor or sufferer—why me? Why did this outbreak occur here at this time? This is the kind of question that may keep a public health official awake at night, wondering what he could have done to prevent the outbreak. In terms of the allegorical painting by William Blake of Satan smiting Job with boils (Figure 1.1), the microbiological meso-scale question is 'What sort of boils are these?', the macro-question to God or Satan is 'Why is this happening?', and the micro-scale question is that of Job: 'Why me?'

What is meant by an emerging disease? It is a socially constructed concept par excellence—some would say it is a cynical social construct for the purpose of raising funds from governments. However, it is an acknowledgement that infections will break out and that there is an element of the unexpected about when and where this will happen.

The concept of 'emerging infections' is a refutation of the view, strongly expressed two decades ago in the London School of Hygiene & Tropical Medicine (LSHTM) as elsewhere, that in developed countries infectious disease was a thing of the past. That this was a fallacy is evident, but it also reflects some newer insights. The picture with which I grew up professionally was one of endemic, high-transmission diseases that needed controlling, plus epidemic diseases which came and went, often in cycles driven by acquired immunity at population level. In addition, there were a few infections driven by partially effective control measures from endemic to epidemic patterns, sometimes with emergence of new clinical problems and disabilities: among these poliomyelitis was the striking example. In this world there was no role for genetic change nor for genetic variation in the pathogen. The extraordinary series of studies carried out at LSHTM by Topley and Greenwood throughout the 1930s using mice and *Salmonella typhimurium*, strange though they may seem to the present reader, showed beyond reasonable doubt that successive epidemics of mouse typhoid were not due to pathogen variation but to the interplay of an unchanging pathogen and of immunity and demographic processes in the mice (Greenwood *et al*, 1936). Occam's razor, that is, the idea that hypotheses should be as simple as possible, plus the adequacy of these processes to explain epidemics, left no need for genetic change. As in the rest of biology, ecological (and epidemiological) change was viewed as being on a very different time-scale from genetic change, and so the latter could be effectively ignored as a major determinant of changes in the pattern of infectious diseases. This is something of a caricature since the importance of antigenic change in influenza was already well known, and myxomatosis was being studied by Fenner (Fenner and Radcliff, 1965), but it does reflect the overall ethos of the time, especially in the UK where genetics had grown up more separately from the rest of biology than in the USA. Everything that has happened since around 1950 has tended to show that genetic and ecological time are not so different, and that, especially in micro-organisms, genetic change can take place rapidly with major consequences for the public health.

Recent advances have not only shown how genetic change plays a key role in the emergence or re-emergence of many diseases, but have also provided methods for the investigation of epidemics of a far greater sophistication than before, so that we have both an awareness of emerging diseases, and better tools with which to understand them and to plan control measures.

There are therefore three questions to be considered in relation to 'emerging diseases':

- What are emerging diseases?
- What are the processes leading to emergence?
- Can we stop them?

The first is a taxonomic question, although there is more to it than that. It is a necessary preamble to the second question, which is the epidemiological and pathogenetic question—the field covered in this chapter. The third question is that of public health which combines action, practicability and cost with science.

Several people have tried to define emerging diseases: initially as a way to escape from the difficulties raised by describing a disease as 'new', and then to classify the different forms of emergence. This is useful as it also points to some features of disease emergence. Thus, Grmek (1993) suggests five types of historical emergence of an infection, which in simple terms are:

1. Diseases newly recognized as entities.
2. Diseases not noticed until quantitative or qualitative changes occurred in their manifestations.
3. Diseases that did not previously exist in a particular region.
4. Diseases that previously existed in animal but not human populations.
5. Completely new diseases.

At first sight this is orderly and complete. But careful consideration reveals that many emerging diseases have elements of several of these categories: cholera may spread to a new area, particularly when a new strain has developed, and show new features. HIV has had features of categories 5, 3, 2, 1 and maybe even 4 at different stages of its emergence. Perhaps this classification has two limitations. First, it does not pay sufficient attention to genetic plasticity. Infraspecific shift in the genetic structure of pathogens may be a prerequisite for or concomitant of other categories of emergence and may be crucial in the process. Second, most emergence of disease probably requires a group of changes, some intrinsic to the pathogen, others in the environment or in human behaviour, so that not one but several changes underlie the emergence of infections.

In a few situations where public health measures have been applied to reduce transmission, or where the environment has altered to produce that effect, a clinical problem has emerged paradoxically due to a shift of age-incidence away from infancy or the period of maternal immunity. This happened to polio 40 years ago, and this may also be a consequence of a reduction in malaria transmission in holoendemic areas. But this process is rarely clear-cut, tends to be transient (as transmission soon improves further or slips back) and can easily be given too much attention. Discussions about whether attempts to reduce transmission will be a waste of effort, so far as disease is concerned, are more appropriate than fears of making things worse, except when considering the frequency of revaccination against infections.

Far more problems result from the decline of public health interventions. These are usually long-continued, inconvenient, and their very success makes them politically unpopular: why spend large sums on preventing a disease that nobody has experienced? They are also often measures outside the health care sector and therefore specially vulnerable to economy cuts in departments other than health, which may be paying for them but have little professional understanding of them. Even without this difficulty there are instances of the collapse of public health measures having very bad consequences. For example, in Eastern Europe the virtual collapse of public health has led to diphtheria outbreaks, and also to the spread of malaria in southern areas.

What do we mean by a truly new disease? First, do we mean disease (objectively demonstrable illness in people) or do we mean infection? If the latter, where does a truly new infection come from? If we exclude Hoyle and Wickramasinghe's (1987) view that outer space is the source, and if we are uncomfortable about the idea of spontaneous generation, then the new infection must be derived from another microbe by mutation, transformation, or other genetic change. The role of plasmids gives plausibility to a much broader range of such events than was once believed and the diversity of genetic exchange needs better understanding by public health workers and not just by specialist microbiologists.

It is important that the current picture of emerging disease is put in proper perspective: the idea that the problems are much worse today than in the past is probably wrong. It is harder for any disease outbreak to pass unnoticed (or information to be suppressed) than was the case in the past—information spreads more easily, and, indeed, the media may amplify an outbreak out of all reasonable proportion, as with the 'flesh-eating-bug' story of the UK newspapers. Many disease epidemics and outbreaks in remote places were previously neglected—a yellow fever epidemic in a remote part of Ethiopia in the 1950s that killed 50 000 people, was not known about until it was over. Human memory is short, so that the resurgence of yaws in Ghana or of malaria in South Asia some years after highly effective control activities, gives the impression of things being worse even though there were and are far fewer cases than in the pre-control period. Failed attempts at eradication particularly give this impression.

In some infections, a relatively sophisticated system of antigenic variation has evolved, ensuring recurrence. At the level of an individual host, African trypanosomes have evolved the most precise system; at the population level the production of intermittent epidemics by genetic change is best seen in influenza, which in this century must have been responsible for both the greatest number of deaths in an epidemic and for most infectious morbidity worldwide. Although Ewald (1994) has put forward plausible theoretical reasons for the emergence of the 1918 pandemic strain in the Western European theatre of trench warfare, pandemics of influenza usually come from China, and Webster (1993) has suggested convincingly that this results from the intensive rearing of pigs and ducks alongside each other in rural China. At least 14 influenza sub-types are found in birds, and it seems likely that mixing of avian and human strains, with genetic reassortment, takes place in pigs, which can be infected with all these, though other candidate hosts for mixing include horses and some aquatic mammals.

The history of world exploration amply documents the terrible consequences of specific pathogens encountering naive populations: syphilis to Europe in 1493 (Guerra, 1993); measles and other acute viral diseases to Polynesia; Oroya fever among visitors to the Andes and tuberculosis among American Indians. As the

Table 1.1 Factors suggested as being responsible for the emergence of diseases

Factors	Bacteria ($n = 17$)	Viruses ($n = 28$)	Parasites ($n = 11$)	Combined ($n = 56$)
Recognition	8	7	1	18
Genetic change	4	2	1	8
Immunosuppression	3	0	8	12
Drug resistance	0	0	1	1
Public health deterioration	0	4	1	6
Technology change	2	5	1	9
Environmental change	3	13	5	24
Food hygiene	1	1	1	3
Human behaviour change	1	6	2	10
Travel	0	5	3	9
Total no. of factors	22	43	24	89%

Calculated from data in Lederberg *et al*, 1992. Note that the number of micro-organisms is less than the number of factors as sometimes two were mentioned for one disease

human populations of the world have become less isolated, this cause of emerging diseases has decreased and it is perhaps only among the most isolated tribal groups of the Amazon basin that this form of emergence is likely in the future.

Factors leading to emergence

Some sense of the determinants of emergence may be obtained from the careful American review of the problem of emerging diseases in which some 56 emerging infections are listed: 17 bacteria, 28 viruses and 11 animal parasites (Lederberg *et al*, 1992). Some 89 factors are suggested as responsible for their emergence and Table 1.1 lists these, by agent type, in 10 categories. It is noticeable that 18% of the factors are given as 'recognition'. Indeed, 'recognition' accounts for 36% of emergences among the bacterial infections. Such 'emergence' is not necessarily on the debit side—it may amount to discovering an infective cause for a condition previously not causally understood. The demonstration of *Helicobacter* as the cause of peptic ulcer is a clear example. Immunosuppression is an emergence factor in 11% of cases, predominantly among the parasitic protozoa where eight emergent pathogens have been identified. Presumably these were present previously in human populations at a subclinical level, as models of highly efficient transmission combined with quiet co-existence with their hosts. Viral emergence was ascribed to ecological changes particularly often, as in agricultural developments, since many of the emerging viral diseases are zoonoses, or were zoonoses initially.

Rather than viewing diseases individually, this chapter now considers types of process leading to disease emergence, with some illustrations, as a basis for rationally coping with or, better, preventing these diseases. Emergence in each

Table 1.2 Role of day care centres in the emergence of diseases among children in the USA

	Children in day care centres	Controls
(A) Relative risk of diseases		
Diarrhoea	2.2–3.5	1
Otitis media	2.0–3.6	1
Invasive pneumococcal disease	4–36	1
Respiratory infections	3.4	1
(B) Second-order consequences		
Use of antibiotics—relative risk of use	3	
Eight-week period prevalence of use (%)	36	8
Mean days of use	19.5	4.6
(C)Third-order consequences		
Point prevalence of resistance to trinethoprim	31	6

Data taken from Holmes *et al*, 1996. In (A) and (B) controls were children at home. In (C) controls were children from a well child clinic

situation requires genetic or environmental change, or both, often linked to human behavioural change. Often, but not always, several changes may occur together, while some factors, such as travel from one place to another, have behavioural, cultural, demographic and environmental change aspects.

Behavioural and cultural processes

Human behaviour and culture, especially as they affect the 'pattern of living', greatly affect disease emergence. Anthony McMichael deals with the large-scale demographic aspects (this volume, chapter 2), but smaller-scale patterns of crowding in communities and dwellings may have a large effect: an early work by Greenwood (1935) was aptly entitled *Epidemics and Crowd-diseases*. Patterns of living and economy affect sexual behaviour, with great consequences for HIV and sexually transmitted diseases.

Behavioural and culture change effects are reflected in the increase of bacterial disease related to mothers in the USA going out to work and needing to have their young children looked after during the day at 'care centres' set up for the purpose, or as part of a group looked after by a neighbour. Holmes and colleagues (1996) have shown a rise in disease risk (Table 1.2A), in the consequential use of antibiotics for treatment or prophylaxis (Table 1.2B) and in the subsequent prevalence of antibiotic resistance in the commensal bacteria of such children (Table 1.2C).

Food-related behaviour affects disease emergence profoundly. Quite subtle changes in food production may affect disease, for example the use of polythene bags for mushroom transport led to the emergence of clostridial toxins. However, the real disasters related to food hygiene have resulted more from risky behaviour or simply bad public health, for example, reducing the criteria for feed processing for cattle and ignoring the evolutionary likelihood that cattle, as herbivores, might not be adequately protected against the risks of carnivory. Considered from this point of view the emergence of the new form of Creutzfeldt–Jakob disease (CJD) is not surprising. The pathogenic strain of *Escherichia coli* strain O157 raises fascinating questions about its origins, how far it is a new organism and why it has become so much more common (Armstrong *et al*, 1996), but the recent outbreaks of disease due to O157 in the UK have been due to violation of basic health precautions of a traditional type. The emergence of disease involving these types of commercially driven behavioural change that involve cutting corners and lowering standards owes something to ruthless pressure to lower costs and to competition without limits. Robust public health barriers are still needed.

Similar factors apply in part to the emergence of water-borne diseases, which are due less to novelty of pathogens than to inadequate basic water treatment. Pressure on sources and neglect of slow sand filtration have led to the emergence of giardiasis and cryptosporidiosis with relatively chlorine-resistant cysts. Peri-urban population pressure in Africa has led to a semi-rural pattern of life at high population density. Plots are small, and when the longstanding conventions of keeping 30 metres between pit latrine and well or borehole are observed on one plot, it often brings the well much closer than 30 metres to a neighbour's latrine! Yet another set of problems result from miscalculation of relative environmental risks, where the media may drive popular perceptions of environmental concerns that have been inappropriately formulated. Adversarial reporting may exaggerate particular risks, with divergence between popular and expert opinion. The most tragic example was in Peru where stories about water chlorination and cancer risk had, completely unjustifiably, led to chlorination being discontinued by several Peruvian water supply managers, so greatly facilitating the spread of epidemic cholera.

New technology may bring more unexpected new diseases. The waters of air-conditioning systems and other warm water devices that create aerosols have shown a remarkable ability to propagate and disperse *Legionella* in localized epidemics (Breiman, 1996).

Conventional environmental changes

Land and water resource developments may lead to the emergence of vector-borne diseases, since most vectors breed in such habitats. There are several clear examples of this process. The introduction of irrigation in arid parts of India has led to malaria epidemics. But such relationships vary locally, and irrigation of the Sahel and other areas of Africa with seasonal malaria has variable effects—in Mali, Burkina Faso and Burundi malaria has not become worse. In The Gambia, the development of irrigated rice was followed by a second anopheline mosquito peak, in the dry season, but no malaria occurred during this second peak, for reasons that remain uncertain (Lindsay *et al*, 1991). (See also Gomes, this volume, chapter 7.)

Other vector-borne disease emergence may relate well to the ecology. For example, Japanese encephalitis in Sarawak is due to the association of rice fields that breed the *Culex* vector and attract the water bird reservoir hosts, pig populations that act as amplifier hosts for the virus, and people (Simpson *et al*, 1976). On the other hand, introduction of irrigated rice in Western Kenya on the Kano plains had little effect on arbovirus activity (Johnson *et al*, 1977). Epidemics of Rift Valley fever in Senegal have been associated with intermittent inundation of large shallow dry basin areas that contained vast deposited numbers of eggs of the *Aedes* vector (Fontenille *et al*, 1995).

Attempts to predict the local emergence of infections have been only partially successful. When Lake Volta in Ghana was created by damming the river, a schistosomiasis risk was anticipated but the intermediate host snail was of a different species, and many had expected intestinal rather than the urinary schistosomiasis that occurred. Similarly, one could have anticipated a schistosomiasis increase following the construction of a dam on the Senegal river but not the explosive outbreak of *Schistosoma mansoni* that took place at Richard Toll.

Great increases in malaria may be associated with the process of deforestation in Asia and South America, though the disease incidence may fall once the forests have completely gone. Reafforestation may increase the risk again from malaria (Gomes, this volume, chapter 7), and in the north-east of the USA, Lyme disease, due to a tick-borne spirochaete, has emerged due to housing and woodland becoming closely interspersed, with an increase in wild deer populations.

Zoonoses have been a major category of emerging diseases, as was well documented by Pavlovsky (1966) in a series of expeditions to the areas of the eastern and southern USSR settled following the Russian revolution. New settlements in the taiga suffered outbreaks of Russian spring–summer encephalitis carried by ticks, whereas new territories in Soviet Central Asia were troubled by rural cutaneous leishmaniasis and plague as the settlers were brought into contact with extensive burrows of colonial gerbils which acted as reservoir for these infections. Subsequently, Audy (1968) in Malaysia showed how jungle settlements led to the emergence of mite-borne typhus or tsutsugamushi fever and he laid emphasis on ecological interfaces or ecotones as a source of hazard. The forest–agricultural ecotone today is a key area for the emergence of multidrug-resistant malaria in Thailand, where smugglers, illicit miners and loggers, and Karen refugees are brought into contact with highly efficient vector anophelines.

In zoonoses which pass into the larger human communities there are often vectors or hosts at the ecotones which have particular importance. For the transition from jungle yellow fever of monkeys transmitted by *Aedes africanus* in the high forest to urban yellow fever spread between people by the peri-domestic *Ae. aegypti*, there is a need for the 'shuttle' vector in Africa *Ae. simpsoni* that can fly across the ecotone. For Ebola fever to spread to cause epidemics it appears that sometimes a sick monkey cut up by the people may act as a shuttle host. In other cases, such as the South American and African arenaviruses (Junin, Machupo, Lassa), changes in agricultural practice bring people into regular contact with the reservoir rodents rather than their cycles of transmission remaining separate.

Travel

While environments may change in themselves, travel and migration bring people and other organisms into new environments, leading to either spread of disease to new places or emergence of increased transmission. It requires both a historical event and ecological receptivity in the new habitat. Although there is substantial global mixing of pathogens as a result of travel, there remain situations—most notably the absence of yellow fever from Asia—where absence of disease may be a historical accident (it could for yellow fever also be due to prior existence of interfering viruses). Disease vectors may often have failed to reach an area. The emergence of epidemic falciparum malaria in Brazil in the 1930s was due to the establishment of *Anopheles gambiae* imported from Africa.

Relative isolation may also matter. The accumulating work on sexual networks and HIV suggest limited sexual mixing between, for example, specific urban and rural groups in South West Uganda.

Conclusions

This short review of a huge topic points to several conclusions. Local epidemiological processes leading to disease emergence are complex and often particular to a specific place and disease. While ‘unprovoked’ genetic change in pathogens may occur, except in a few specialised micro-organisms, such as influenza virus, this is not the commonest cause of emergence. Mixing of populations and environmental change are more important. Change is inevitable, but the more hazardous consequences of such change are often predictable and avoidable. Public health measures of the past were solid and robust and care is needed before they are relaxed. Marginalization, whether geographical or economic, increases vulnerability. While problems of genetic change are increasingly acute as the use of chemotherapy and pesticides is great, opportunities for analysis of genetic change are incomparably greater than a few years ago. To use Hutchinson’s metaphor, emergence involves changes in both the ecological theatre and the evolutionary play (Hutchinson, 1965). More prosaically, it often involves basic local failures of public health practice as well as more scientifically fascinating topics.

In summary, the proximate and local causes of tomorrow’s epidemics may perhaps be described in terms of five people who lived within two blocks of LSHTM, where this Public Health Forum was held, or are involved in the origins of the LSHTM. They result from changes in:

- *behaviour and culture*, as represented by the writer and novelist Virginia Woolf
- *economic pressures*, possibly involving migrations, as represented by the economist Maynard Keynes, who shared a house just beyond Malet Street
- *environmental change*, as represented by John Constable, who painted the rural environment but lived almost on the site of LSHTM
- *genetic and evolutionary changes in pathogens*, represented by Charles Darwin who lived one block to the north, and
- *biological vector changes*, and *variations in public health practice*, as represented by Ronald Ross.

Their location may remind us that emergence is usually not due to a single factor, that the predominant factors may vary over time, and that often local factors are superimposed on a larger-scale change that may have been occurring gradually.

References

Armstrong GL, Hollingsworth J, Morris JG. Emerging food borne pathogens: *Escherichia coli* O157:H7 as a model of entry of a new pathogen into the food supply of the developed world. *Epidemiologic Reviews*, 1996; **18**: 29–51

Audy JR. *Red Mites and Typhus*. London: Athlone Press, 1968

Breiman RF. Impact of technology in the emergence of infectious diseases. *Epidemiologic Reviews*, 1996; **18**: 4–9

Ewald PW. *Evolution of Infectious Disease*. Oxford: Oxford University Press, 1994

Fenner F, Ratcliffe FN. *Myxomatosis*. Cambridge: Cambridge University Press, 1965

Fontenille D, Traore-Lamizana M, Zeller H, Mondo M, Diallo M, Digoutte JP. Short report: Rift Valley fever in western Africa: isolations from Aedes mosquitoes during an interepizootic period. *American Journal of Tropical Medicine and Hygiene*, 1995; **52**: 403–404

Greenwood M. *Epidemics and Crowd-diseases: An Introduction to the Study of Epidemiology*. London: Williams and Norgate, 1935

Greenwood M, Hill AB, Topley WWC, Wilson J. *Experimental Epidemiology*. Medical Research Council Special Reports Series 209, 1936

Grmek MD. Le concept de maladie émergente. *Pubblicazioni della Stazione Zoologica di Napoli. Section II: History and Philosophy of the Life Sciences (London)*, 1993; **15**: 281–296

Guerra F. The European–American exchange. *Pubblicazioni della Stazione Zoologica di Napoli. Section II: History and Philosophy of the Life Sciences (London)*, 1993; **15**: 313–328

Holmes SJ, Morrow AL, Pickering LK. Child-care practices: effects of social change in the epidemiology of infectious diseases and antibiotic resistance. *Epidemiologic Reviews*, 1996; **18**: 10–28

Hoyle F, Wickramasinghe NC. Influenza viruses and comets. *Nature*, 1987; **327**: 664

Hutchinson GE. *The Ecological Theater and the Evolutionary Play*. New Haven, CT: Yale University Press, 1965

Johnson BK, Shockley P, Chanas AC *et al*. Arbovirus isolations from mosquitoes: Kano Plain, Kenya. *Transactions of the Royal Society of Tropical Medicine and Hygiene*, 1977; **71**: 518–521

Lederberg J, Shope RE, Oaks SC. *Emerging Infections: Microbial Threats to Health in the United States*. Washington: National Academy Press, 1992

Lindsay SW, Wilkins HA, Zieler HA, Daly RJ, Petrarca V, Byass P. Ability of *Anopheles gambiae* mosquitoes to transmit malaria during the dry and wet seasons in an area of irrigated rice cultivation in The Gambia. *Journal of Tropical Medicine and Hygiene*, 1991; **94**: 313–324

Pavlovsky EN. *Natural Nidality of Transmissible Diseases.* Urbana, IL: University of Illinois Press, 1966

Simpson DI, Smith CE, Marshall TF *et al.* Arbovirus infections in Sarawak: the role of the domestic pig. *Transactions of the Royal Society of Tropical Medicine and Hygiene*, 1976; **70**: 66–72

Webster RG. Influenza. In: Morse SS, *Emerging Viruses.* New York: Oxford University Press, 1993, pp 37–45

Discussion

T. Jacob John

Christian Medical College, Vellore, India

David Bradley has illustrated with several examples how relatively minor local changes can increase the risk of developing certain infectious diseases. India provides several recent examples of how certain changes, man-made or otherwise, have brought about unexpected outbreaks of infectious diseases. There are logical explanations for many of these episodes, and by understanding them it should be possible to anticipate the consequences of other similar changes in behaviour or the physical environment.

Emerging infections in India

Typhoid fever

South India recently experienced a large outbreak of typhoid fever which started in 1991 and lasted nearly two years (Jesudason *et al*, 1996). This was part of a nationwide epidemic of enormous magnitude; the economic loss due to it has not been calculated. The strain of *Salmonella typhi* responsible for the epidemic was resistant to chloramphenicol, ampicillin and co-trimoxazole, the three standard antimicrobials used in the treatment of typhoid fever. This multiple-drug resistance (MDR) was plasmid-mediated. *S. typhi* is an exclusive human parasite. Typhoid fever is endemic in all parts of India, so why did this MDR organism cause the epidemic? Infected persons may have amplified transmission as a result of a delay in treatment with a fluoroquinolone to which the strain of *S. typhi* was sensitive.

Dengue in Delhi

In 1996 there was a large outbreak of dengue haemorrhagic fever in Delhi. Two decades ago dengue did not occur in Delhi, but during the past decade, dengue has become endemic, with annual post-monsoon outbreaks. It is believed that the vector mosquitoes (*Aedes egypti*) breed in household desert coolers, which have increased in number some 500-fold in the past 10 years. People are supposed to empty the water from their coolers as monsoon breaks in; if they do not, the stagnant water that remains is an excellent breeding ground for the vector mosquitoes.

Malaria

The resurgence of malaria in India is partly due to an increase in the anopheline vector mosquitoes as a result of an increase in irrigated agriculture. Owing to inadequate primary health care, malarial parasites are allowed to persist in people, resulting in a vicious spiral (Sharma, 1996).

Plague, leptospirosis and cholera

Although plague is endemic in India, until recently no human cases had been recognized since the 1960s. Surveillance of the sylvatic foci of plague was stopped. In the Beed district of central India, an earthquake occurred in 1993. In Mamla village in the affected area, people shifted to shelters with light roofs, but continued to use their houses for storing grains. This resulted in a massive increase in the population of rodents, which appear to have been a major factor in the outbreak of suspected bubonic plague reported in 1994 (Saxena and Verghese, 1996). The same year there was an outbreak of suspected pneumonic plague in Surat city in Western India. Confirmation of the aetiology of this outbreak took several months and in the intervening period there was considerable uncertainty about the nature of the illness. Although the source of the outbreak was confirmed finally using a polymerase chain reaction for the detection of *Yersinia pestis* DNA in stored autopsy tissues, the opportunity to examine the origin or modes of transmission was lost (Panda *et al*, 1996).

There has been a resurgence of leptospirosis in southern India since 1987 (Panda *et al*, 1996). Although the exact ecological changes that have brought about this rise are not known, they are likely to be related to agricultural practices and rodent bionomics.

The recent history of cholera in India is intriguing. Although Bengal is the main endemic focus for cholera, it was in South India that *Vibrio cholerae* 0139 emerged as a new pathogen (John, 1996). Many experts believe that *V. cholerae* 01 and 0139 are aquatic organisms, growing and surviving in the algal plankton. The changes that brought about the emergence of this new organism remain unsolved.

Where do parasites come from?

Each infectious agent has its own unique biological properties, ecological niche, transmission characteristics and disease potential. Therefore generalizations can be hazardous but some can be made. Infectious agents have certain specific requirements for multiplication and survival—the amplification system. Different infectious agents have different pathways of transmission—the transmission system. After the agent has reached the host there are many factors which determine whether the person becomes infected or not and whether infection causes disease or not—the parasite–host interaction system. Control of infectious diseases can be targeted at any of these systems or at a combination of more than one. By the same token, local changes may influence any one of these component systems, resulting in more microbes, more transmission or more disease.

Local changes influencing the rise of infectious diseases

The two models presented do not describe the influence of local changes in the rise of infectious diseases, but they help us in understanding why local changes may influence infectious diseases. They also help us in predicting what local changes might do to infectious agents and also help to define remedial measures to counter the ill effects of changes.

In the case of the Indian outbreak of MDR typhoid fever, the delay in bactericidal therapy enhanced the amplification system. In the case of dengue and malaria, local changes had affected both the amplification and transmission systems. In 1994, an outbreak of cholera in Vellore town coincided with a break in chlorination of the water supply due to an administrative error. As soon as chlorination was resumed the outbreak ceased. Here the local change affected exclusively the transmission system.

The story of Bolivian haemorrhagic fever is well known. In the San Joaquin Valley region, a rodent virus, now called Machupo, caused an epidemic with a very high fatality rate. The sequence of events that led to this outbreak were deforestation, corn cultivation, invasion of the displaced rodents into human habitations and infection of humans with the virus by inhalation or ingestion. The lesson here, in the plague story, and in the case of Hantavirus outbreaks in different parts of the world, is that rodents must be kept under watch and under control. Rodents are involved even in the emergence of Lyme borreliosis. The ticks (*Ixodes dammini*) have two hosts: a rodent in the larval stage and the deer in the adult stage. Reforestation in many regions in the USA has resulted in an increase in the deer population, and in their parasitic ticks. Thus, contact between ticks and humans increased and the ticks transmitted the spirochaete to humans.

Conclusion

When we knowingly or unknowingly alter the ecology of our environment, the resultant changes are sometimes unpredictable. When such changes affect the amplification or the transmission systems of any infectious agent, then they may lead to an increased incidence of the disease.

The unpredictability principle also deserves our attention. We do not know what ecological pressures led to the emergence of *V. cholerae* 0139; that it appeared in South India compounds the mystery. The MDR plasmid in *S. typhi* could be explained as a consequence of the overuse of antibiotics; such plasmids are known to be transferred across species among *Enterobacteriaceae*.

For detecting local changes and their consequences in relation to infectious diseases, six items deserve constant monitoring everywhere. They are food hygiene, quality of drinking water, vector bionomics, rodents and their parasites, locally prevalent diseases and antimicrobial susceptibility/resistance patterns of relevant pathogens. Eternal vigilance is the price of freedom from epidemics.

References

Jesudason MV, John R, John TJ. The concurrent prevalence of chloramphenicol sensitive and multi-drug resistant *Salmonella typhi* in Vellore, S. India. *Epidemiology and Infection*, 1996; **116**: 225–227

John TJ. Emerging and re-emerging bacterial pathogens in India. *Indian Journal of Medical Research*, 1996; **103**: 4–18

Panda SK, Nanda SK, Ghosh A *et al.* The 1994 plague epidemic in India: molecular diagnosis and characterisation of *Yersinia pestis* isolates from Surat and Beed. *Current Science*, 1996; **71**: 794–799

Saxena VK, Verghese T. Ecology of flea-transmitted zoonotic infection in village Mamla, District Beed. *Current Science*, 1996; **71**: 800–802

Sharma VP. Re-emergence of malaria in India. *Indian Journal of Medical Research*, 1996; **103**: 26–45

2
The influence of historical and global changes upon the patterns of infectious diseases

Anthony J. McMichael

London School of Hygiene & Tropical Medicine, UK

Throughout recorded and prerecorded history, humankind has encountered new and resurgent infectious diseases. We are surrounded and inhabited by microbes. Theirs is a world of extraordinary and rapid genetic lability, of freely exchanged genetic material (unrestrained by the formalities of sexual reproduction) and of agile ecological opportunism. Over a long period microbes have honed their adaptive skills to deal with nutrient shortages, hostile immune systems and antibiotics. Evolutionarily, humans are newcomers.

Appreciation of the ceaseless interplay between human ecology and the microbial world requires consideration of four macroscopic perspectives:

1. The co-evolution, over many millennia, of infectious agents and the human species.
2. The historical confluence of disease pools between major civilizations.
3. The global changes in today's world that are influencing the range and incidence of infectious diseases.
4. The continuing role of social, economic and political conditions on the pattern of infectious diseases.

Infectious diseases: an evolutionary history

The eminent historian, William McNeill, has suggested that human cultural evolution has repeatedly disturbed the biological equilibrium between humans and microbes but that, in the fullness of time, natural forces act to re-establish equilibrium (McNeill, 1976). Twice, humans have prised themselves partially free

New and Resurgent Infections: Prediction, Detection and Management of Tomorrow's Epidemics.
Edited by B. Greenwood and K. De Cock.

of the heavy burden of infection—first, around 100 000 years ago when the modern human species began to disperse out of parasitically dense Africa; second, around 100 years ago when modern ideas on the causes and ways of preventing infectious diseases emerged. In each case, subsequent developments have pulled us back into a closer relationship with infectious agents. The second of those two re-equilibration processes underlies the contemporary interest in the 'emergence and resurgence' of infectious diseases in the late twentieth century.

Humans have both 'heirloom' and 'acquired' infections (Karlen, 1995). The heirloom infections are presumed to have been handed on to early hominids from primate ancestors. Free-living primates are today infected with infections such as malaria, hepatitis, yaws and herpes simplex infection. Heirloom infections include the commensal bacteria that flourish in mouths, throats, stomachs and intestines. They also include several persistent, mildly debilitating, helminths (tapeworms, pinworms, hookworms, etc.) which, through hard-won evolutionary adaptation, have learnt to down-regulate the host's immunological response. Early hominids probably carried several of these non-immunogenic parasitic helminths, maintained by unhurried transmission between successive generations. Other heirloom infectious agents probably included chronic low-impact viruses (such as Epstein–Barr virus and cytomegalovirus) and some relatively benign forms of staphylococci, streptococci and enteric coliform bacteria.

In later millennia, human demographic and cultural changes provided a succession of new opportunities for new microbes. The mutant microbial strains that occupied these unfolding ecological niches have become humankind's 'acquired' infections. The process continues today, as the HIV/AIDS pandemic dramatically affirms. HIV is just one more instance of this perennial traffic of microbial and molecular 'hopefuls' across the species barrier. Most of these mutant hopefuls fail; a few succeed—some spectacularly.

The initial change from tree-dwelling to ground-dwelling that took place around 5–6 million years ago in eastern Africa—the acknowledged evolutionary cradle of the hominid line—must have brought a radical change in the microbial parasitic environment for the newly upright-walking australopithecine hominids. Soil-dwelling hookworms were encountered. So, too, was an unfamiliar constellation of mosquitoes.

As global cooling accelerated dramatically, from around 2.5 million years ago, australopithecines began to be superseded by the emergent bigger-brained *Homo* genus. The use of animal skins for rudimentary clothing and shelter, and a heightened reliance on eating meat in an increasingly cold and arid world, must have brought further contact with various food-borne helminths and bacteria.

Because human groups remained small, sporadically encountered contagious infections could not sustain themselves as endemic, acute infections. Then, around 15 000 BP, a momentous change occurred. The last long glaciation began to recede and Earth entered a long, but erratic, warming phase (approximately 5°C in 5000 years). The fossil record shows that this resulted in climatic stresses upon many species of edible animals and wild plant foods, thus depleting the food supplies of humans. In low-to-middle latitudes, humans responded, of necessity, by learning to grow plants and herd animals. Slowly, effective techniques to do this evolved, food supplies increased, and consequently so did human numbers. Living became more settled and less nomadic. Villages, towns and, later, cities appeared.

Human populations were thus transformed progressively into an auspicious culture medium for infectious agents. A new and profound equilibrium between microbe and human became possible. There was now a sufficiently large and dense human population for the sustained circulation of infectious agents, including those that cause a lasting immunity in infected survivors. Human settlements were pervaded by their own accumulated waste and excreta, enabling the efficient recycling of infectious agents. Furthermore, the potential of infection from animals was increased because of the herding and domestication of animals. Likewise, the clearing of land for agriculture put humans into closer contact with disturbed ecosystems, from which they encountered new mosquito-borne, tick-borne and rodent-borne protozoans, bacteria and viruses.

The combination of human agriculture, animal husbandry and early urbanization, from around 6000–8000 years ago, created the conditions needed for sustained endemic infections and for periodic outbreaks of epidemic infectious disease. The earliest urban populations of half a million persons or more occurred in Mesopotamian Sumeria around 5000 years ago. Such populations would have been large enough to sustain diseases such as measles. Even so, the historical record is sparse; the best evidence of measles from Sumeria is a stone inscription describing epidemics and invoking the Goddess of Epidemics.

A few infective agents, such as the yellow fever virus, may have infected these early human civilizations directly. Others, of zoonotic origin, became human pathogens via mutational change that enabled them to cross the species divide. Thus arose many of today's familiar infectious diseases, such as measles and chickenpox (Karlen, 1995). Tuberculosis and smallpox are thought to have been acquired, via mutant microbes, from zoonotic infections in cattle, measles from dogs, influenza from chickens, leprosy from water buffalo and the common cold from horses.

Initially, the impact of these new infectious diseases was probably devastating—because of the immunological and genetic naivety of human populations. Later, as both host and agent co-evolved, many of these infections became common endemic infections that typically infected young persons: measles, smallpox, chickenpox, mumps, whooping cough and others.

The confluence of disease pools between great civilizations

Great civilizations began to appear in western Asia from around 5000 years ago, during the warmer 'Holocene Optimum' period—first in Mesopotamia, then in

Egypt and the Indus Valley. Civilizations in eastern Asia, southern Asia and Mesoamerica followed. Many of them had 'signature' epidemics which, for thousands of years, remained regionally confined (McNeill, 1976). Then, as trade, travel and warfare increased, these boundaries were breached and the ancient pools of infection began to intermix.

Two thousand years ago, the Roman Empire and the Han Dynasty, at the opposite ends of Eurasia, made contact. Epidemiological catastrophe occurred; virulent new plagues ravaged both populations. An eventual super-continental pooling resulted in an uneasy Eurasian equilibrium. The uncompromising process of selective survival in this supra-population resulted in a human stock genetically more able to cope with these infections. Even so, the fourteenth century plague in Europe (the 'Black Death') underscored the incomplete nature of such co-evolutionary adaptation. This unprecedented catastrophe resulted from a combination of intensified caravan trade across the Asian steppes, warfare around the Black Sea ports, a deteriorating climate at the end of the 'Mediaeval warm' associated with impaired crop yields in Europe, and some corresponding climatic disturbances in the Central Asian heartland of the rodent reservoir of plague. Some commentators have also invoked the beginnings of the breakdown in the feudal system as a contributory factor (Epstein, this volume, chapter 3). The plague arrived in the Mediterranean region in 1346; two years later it swept into Britain.

In the fifteenth century, human contact across the Atlantic occurred. As a result, immunologically naive native populations of the Americas were devastated by European infections and may have sent back several in return (referred to by historians as 'the Columbian Exchange'). Meanwhile, European armies, engaged in a profusion of religious and territorial wars, began exchanging syphilis, typhus, the mysterious 'English Sweating Sickness' and other infections. Later, in the Australasian and Pacific region, remote aboriginal populations were devastated by unfamiliar infectious diseases, in particular measles, introduced by European settlers and invaders.

Enhanced ecological opportunities for infectious agents do not depend exclusively upon human agency. Natural processes ensure continuous exchange of genetic material between bacteria, viruses, plasmids and prophages (Mathieu and Sonea, 1995). For example, the emergence of life-threatening cholera in 1817, the year of the first recorded pandemic, may have followed the insertion of viral DNA from a naturally occurring virus carrying a CTX gene into the *Cholera vibrio* genome, thus enabling the vibrio to produce the potent CTX toxin. Human cultural practices can greatly enhance this exchange and mixing of microbial DNA. A well known example is the DNA recombination that occurs between avian flu viruses that also infect domestic pigs in southern China (Karlen, 1995). This duck–pig farming complex is an efficient source of recombinant flu viruses that then pass into the human population and circulate globally. A similar process may occur in an individual infected by different HIV viral subtypes;

genetic recombination within the host enables more virulent or more infective recombinant HIV subtypes to emerge under the intense selection pressures of immune attack.

The endless ecological and social narrative of human infectious disease continues into modern times. The bovine-to-human link in the UK's current nvCJD outbreak (Smith, this volume, chapter 10), underscores a timeless truth—namely, that the world is full of microbes jostling for supplies of nutrients, energy and molecular building blocks. Occasionally, via the relentless probing processes of natural selection, they discover a new niche in macrobes, human or other. The right mutant microbe in the right place can found a micro-dynasty. It has happened many times before, and will continue to do so in the future.

Global environmental change and infectious disease

During this century, the aggregate environmental impact of human economic enterprise has become so large that it has begun to change some of the world's great biophysical systems (McMichael, 1993a). The composition of the lower and middle atmospheres is changing. The former is likely to cause global climate change (IPCC, 1996); the latter is increasing the amount of ultraviolet radiation reaching Earth's surface. Large-scale changes are becoming more evident in several other major biophysical systems; these include widespread loss of biodiversity, declines in major freshwater aquifers on every continent, and the global dispersion of various non-biodegradable chemical pollutants. These global environmental changes pose various, somewhat unfamiliar, risks to human health (Last, 1993; McMichael, 1993b).

Change in global climate and infectious disease

The UN's Intergovernmental Panel on Climate Change has forecast an average global increase in temperature of around 2°C by 2100 (IPCC, 1996). The IPCC has cautiously concluded that there is now evidence of a discernible human influence upon world climate, a contribution to the almost half-degree centigrade rise in temperature seen over the past three decades.

The anticipated health effects of climate change include alterations in the range and prevalence of vector-borne infectious diseases such as malaria, leishmaniasis and dengue, changes in rates of direct transmission of anthroponotic infections (including food-poisoning and water-borne pathogens) and of zoonotic infections such as rabies and hantavirus (McMichael *et al*, 1996). The vector-borne diseases are of particular interest since the small, cold-blooded vectors that spread diseases such as malaria, dengue fever, yellow fever, trypanosomiasis, the viral encephalitides and schistosomiasis are very sensitive to climatic factors, especially temperature, humidity and the distribution of surface water (Patz *et al*, 1996). Increased mean and minimum temperatures, and altered rainfall, are likely to affect the range, proliferation and behaviour of vector organisms—and the viability and maturation rates of the infectious agents that they carry. Recent observations suggest that ecological changes related to warming are already occurring on all continents. Thus, there has been an upward retreat of mountain glaciers, the migration of alpine plant species to higher altitudes, and the movement of dengue, malaria or their mosquito vectors to higher altitudes (Epstein, 1997).

Malaria

Several recent studies based on predictive mathematical modelling have projected that, under standard global climate change scenarios, the potential geographic range for malaria transmission will expand next century (Martens *et al*, 1995; Martin and Lefebvre, 1995). Approximately 45% of the world's population currently lives in climate-defined zones of *potential* malaria transmission; under anticipated conditions of climate change this would increase to around 60% by the latter part of the next century. Such attempts to model future impacts of climate change at a global level have typically been highly aggregated and they are, therefore, unable to take account of regional and local particularities. More recently, such modelling has been down-scaled as, for example, for malaria in Zimbabwe (Martens, 1997).

Further insight on the relationship between infectious diseases and climate comes from study of the way in which natural fluctuations in climate affect vector-borne infectious diseases. For example, malaria outbreaks in the Thar Desert, western Rajasthan, depend primarily on annual rainfall (Akhtar and McMichael, 1996). The major source of variability in world weather patterns is the 'El Niño Southern Oscillation' (ENSO) process, based in the central Pacific Ocean and driven by interannual variations in the east–west atmospheric pressure gradient. These aperiodic reversals of wind flow, and hence of warm surface waters and moist air across the Pacific, cause droughts at low-to-mid latitudes around the world. ENSO variation accounts for up to 40% of the variation in temperature and rainfall in the Pacific (Hales *et al*, 1996). Several recent studies have shown how ENSO-related temperature and rainfall patterns affect the occurrence of malaria in north-east Pakistan and Sri Lanka (Bouma *et al*, 1994; Bouma and van der Kaay, 1996). Before the introduction of residual insecticides, malaria epidemics in the Punjab typically occurred in high-rainfall years that followed soon after the dry El Niño years (Bouma and van der Kaay, 1995). Rainfall in West Rajasthan in the year following an El Niño event is approximately 40% higher than in the El Niño year and is 50% higher in the 'La Niña' years (i.e. the opposite phase of ENSO) (Bouma and Cox, personal communication).

In much of Europe and North America, the existing levels of public health may suffice to prevent the reintroduction of malaria (at least over the next few decades). Actual increases in malaria in response to climate change are most likely to occur in vulnerable populations currently at the margins of established endemic areas, particularly in the tropical and subtropical regions—for example, those living at altitudes just above the present level of malaria transmission and those living on the edge of towns.

Dengue fever

Dengue fever is the world's most frequent vector-borne viral disease, causing around 100 million cases annually, in tropical and subtropical countries. Dengue has been on the increase in recent decades, particularly in Central and South America—probably because of trends in population mobility, urbanization, poverty, public health infrastructure and regional climatic changes (Gubler and Clark, 1995; Lifson, 1996).

There are multiple influences upon the rapidly changing world map of dengue. The 1990s dengue epidemic in Central America may reflect, in part, the impact of a warmer global climate. Dengue has been occurring at unusually high altitudes in the highlands of some countries. In the 1980s, it began to appear in highlands in Colombia at 2200 metres, and, during a particularly warm summer in Mexico in 1988, at an historically unprecedented altitude of 1700 metres (Herrera-Basto *et al*, 1992).

The sensitivity of dengue transmission to temperature reflects, in part, the smaller size and more frequent biting habits of the adult *Ae. aegypti* mosquitoes at higher temperatures. It also reflects the concomitant decrease in the extrinsic incubation period of the dengue virus—which, for dengue type-2 virus, is 12 days at 30°C versus seven days at 33–34°C. This five-day shortening of the incubation period can yield a three-fold increase in the dengue transmission rate (Patz *et al*, 1996).

Some research on the possible impact of the ENSO climatic variations upon dengue has been done. Within the South Pacific region, which is currently on the fringe of the endemic zone for dengue, outbreaks of dengue fever in island nations during 1970–95 have correlated moderately well with ENSO events ($r = 0.58$; Hales *et al*, 1996).

Cholera

The origins of cholera remain uncertain (Cook, 1996). It may have occurred in classical times, but descriptions and nomenclature are unclear. Severe outbreaks of dehydrating diarrhoeal diseases are recorded in ancient Chinese and Hindu texts. In recent centuries, Asiatic cholera has been one of the most spectacular of the major pestilences—with seven pandemics since 1817. The reason why cholera eventually broke out of its historical base in the Ganges delta remains obscure, although in the preceding centuries it had flared up in South Asia, nurtured by large, dense populations, poor sanitation, extensive areas of surface water, temperatures above 17°C, and high humidity.

The transmission of cholera may be influenced by local variations in climate acting through planktonic populations. Colwell (1996) has reported that differences in the pattern of the south-west monsoon winds between years are accompanied by variations in summer phytoplankton blooms in the north-western Arabian Sea and in the Bay of Bengal and that variations in sea-surface temperature are correlated with the occurrence of cholera in Bangladesh. Scanning electron microscopy indicates that the cholera vibrio can survive beneath the outer lining of various phytoplanktonic organisms in marine and estuarine surface waters and beneath the chitinous sheath of live zooplankton (Islam *et al*., 1994; Huq *et al*., 1995; Colwell, 1996). Thus, planktonic organisms act as a microhabitat, a type of 'vector'. An example of this process may have occurred in early 1991 when coastal algal blooms coincided with the introduction of *V. cholerae* into offshore waters near Lima, Peru (Tamplin and Carrillo-Parodi, 1991). In this complex web of environmental causation, the occurrence of planktonic blooms may have been affected by increased water temperature due to the onset of an ENSO event, nitrogen–phosphorus eutrophication (via wastewater and fertilizer runoff), and reduced algivorous grazing pressure within the overfished marine food web.

There is a possibility of increased spread of cholera in the future as a result of climatic change if rising sea-levels cause an increase in coastal lagoons of brackish water and if interior continental drying causes an increase in brackish waterways.

Loss of biodiversity and infectious diseases

A loss of biodiversity, including changes in the species composition, in habitats, and in predator–prey relationships, can affect human risks of infectious disease in diverse ways. Lyme disease and hantavirus pulmonary syndrome illustrate such processes.

Lyme disease

Lyme disease has 'emerged' over the past quarter-century. It was first identified in the north-eastern United States where it is now an important public health problem. The disease is caused by a spirochaete, *Borrelia burgdorferi*, transmitted by infected Ixodic ticks. Lyme disease also occurs in Europe and across temperate Asia, where it is transmitted via other subspecies of *Ixodes ricinus* ticks (Barthold, 1996). The tick has a complex three-stage life-cycle, and parasitizes various mammalian species, especially rodents and deer. Transmission is influenced by climate because temperature and rainfall affect the geographic range of the intermediate host mammals and the speed of maturation of the immature (larval–nymphal) tick.

In north-east USA the nymphal stage of the tick is infected by feeding on spirochaete-infected white-footed mice. The tick also feeds on other small mammals if they are present, and most of these other mammals do *not* carry the spirochaete. Hence, in impoverished local ecosystems in which the tick-nymphs are obliged to feed on the infected species of mouse, the proportion of infected ticks is much greater than in ecosystems in which ticks have access to a diversity of vertebrates.

Borrelia have a long and complex evolutionary history (Barthold, 1996). The various Borrelian spirochaete species occur in a globalized mosaic across Europe, Asia and North America. Molecular genetics indicate that these different species of spirochaetes evolved within separate ecosystems. Palaeo-archaeological analysis suggests that this was because of the ecologically disruptive effects of the advance and retreat of the last Ice Age, resulting in the creation of many unique and isolated reservoir (vertebrate) habitats for the tick, and allowing the co-evolution of distinct species of both tick and spirochaete. Subsequent genetic mixing of the Borrelian spirochaete species has occurred, as vertebrate hosts and their ticks have intermingled. This process has been amplified greatly, especially between northern and southern hemispheres, by enzootic cycles of borreliosis in seabirds. Thus, over recent millennia, connections between migratory routes and between birds and rodents have globalized the Borrelian spirochaete species. Further perturbation of the environment and influence on enzootic cycles have occurred via human habitation. 'Lyme disease,' says Barthold (1996), 'is an outstanding example of the complex natural history of an infectious disease emerging in the modern world.'

Hantavirus pulmonary syndrome

The prolonged El Niño event of the early 1990s may have potentiated the unexpected outbreak, in south-west USA in May 1993, of the newly recognised zoonotic disease, hantavirus pulmonary syndrome (Duchin *et al*, 1994). Infected mice excrete the hantavirus in their urine which, after drying, produces viral particles easily spread by the wind. This rodent-borne viral infection is often fatal.

In the early 1990s, the climate of south-west USA was unusually dry, causing widespread declines in animal populations, including those of several predator species (snakes and birds) that eat the virus-carrying mice. Subsequently, the ENSO-associated heavy rains of 1993 led to a local greening, including a profusion of pine-nuts and grasshoppers that fuelled a proliferation of well fed mice. This, in turn, provided a rich resource for the hantavirus, and the infection was disseminated in adjoining rodent populations, spreading, during 1993–1996, to 26 States and causing 74 reported deaths.

Interestingly, a recent reassessment of the ephemeral epidemics of the dramatic but mysterious 'English Sweating Sickness' of the sixteenth century concludes that it may have been this same hantaviral disease (Thwaites *et al*, 1997). The scattered rural distribution and the late-summer peak suggest rodent-borne transmission; the absence of exanthematous or haemorrhagic lesions precludes most arbovirus infections.

Antimicrobials in nature

Nature is a rich source of chemical compounds with antimicrobial properties. Historically, one of the great success stories was that of the anti-malarial, quinine, obtained from the bark of the Cinchona tree. Today, there are many other such stories: streptomycin, neomycin, amphotericin and erythromycin—all of which derive from tropical soil fungi. The soil-dwelling bacterium *Bacillus thuringiensis* produces a distinctive toxin, used to control agricultural pests and the blackfly that transmits onchocerciasis.

Land-use patterns

Disruptive changes in patterns of land use in recent decades have led to the appearance of new infections (Wilson, 1995). This is well illustrated by the new haemorrhagic fever viruses that have emerged in South America and elsewhere associated with forest and grassland clearance and with extensive, subsequent, agricultural mono-cropping (Morse, 1993). Extension of forest-fringe malaria is another example of this process (Sawyer, 1993; Gomes, this volume, chapter 7).

Arena and bunya virus infections associated with agricultural extension in South America include the Argentine (Junin virus) haemorrhagic fever, spread by proliferation of infected mice (*Calomyscus callosus*) in pesticide-cleared pampas grasslands, during the 1950s, and new haemorrhagic fevers in eastern Bolivia (Machupo virus) and Brazil (Sabia virus), connected with disturbances of rodent ecology. In the Amazon basin, Oropouche fever has been spread by virus-infected gnats in cacao plantations. Meanwhile, in rural populations in East Asia there have been increases in outbreaks of infection by the Hantaan virus, transmitted by rodents (*Apodemus agrarius*), in rice-fields.

Changes to the hydrological environment may also have an important influence on patterns of infectious diseases. The building of large dams has affected vector-borne infectious diseases. For example, outbreaks of Rift Valley fever occurred in the Nile Valley in 1977 and in Mauritania in 1987 following the damming of major rivers (Karlen, 1995). Construction of the Aswan dam on the Nile River resulted in a seven-fold increase in schistosomiasis. Lymphatic filariasis in the southern Nile Delta has undergone a 20-fold increase in prevalence since the 1960s, primarily due to an increase in breeding sites for the vector mosquito *Culex pipiens* that followed the rise in the water table due to extensions of irrigation. The situation has been exacerbated by pesticide-resistance in mosquitoes associated with heavy pesticide use by local farmers, and by rural-to-urban commuting among farm-workers (Harb *et al*, 1993).

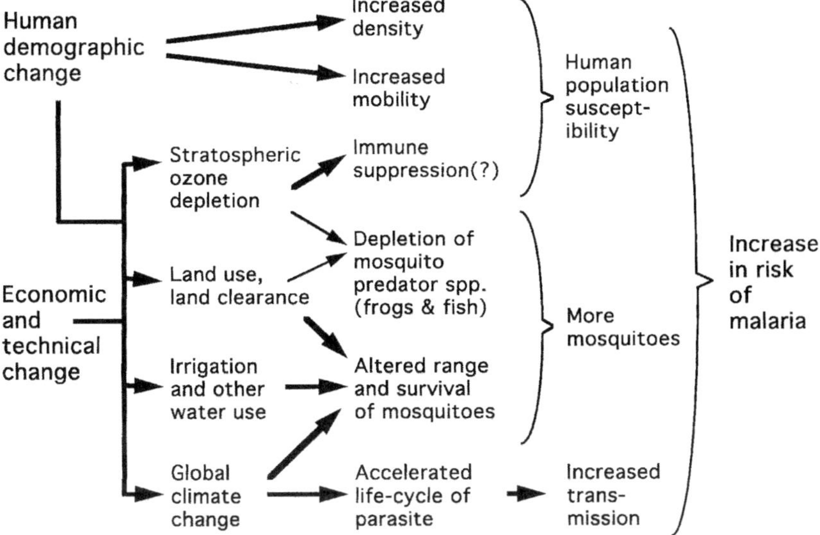

Figure 2.1 Schematic illustration of the multiple influences of co-existent global environmental changes upon the risk of transmission of malaria. The relative importance of specific pathways is not indicated and would vary in different settings. The complexity of the configuration presents a major difficulty to integrated mathematical modelling of multiple interactive environmental influences

Interactive effects of global change processes

Combinations of global environmental changes may greatly enhance risks to health. For example, agricultural production—a major determinant of nutritional status, physical development, and susceptibility to infections in poor countries—is affected by multiple interacting environmental stresses (e.g. climatic change, land degradation, pesticide-induced imbalances in predator–prey relationships, and aquifer depletion). Likewise, it can be anticipated that risks of infectious disease will be affected by a multiplicity of coexistent and intensifying global change processes. Such possibilities are illustrated for malaria in Figure 2.1.

Human social and economic conditions

Changes in social, demographic and economic conditions, including population density, age structure and mobility, all influence patterns of infectious disease (Wilson, 1995). Changes in patterns of commerce and trade may have a similar effect. For example, in the 1980s, shipments of used truck tyres introduced *Aedes albopictus*, the 'tiger' mosquito from East Asia, into the USA and Brazil (Morse, 1993). This mosquito, which transmits dengue in Asia, has now spread regionally and is a potential new vector for dengue and, perhaps, other viruses in the Americas.

Socioeconomic inequalities and poverty exert profound influences on the patterns of infectious diseases (Castilla and Sawyer, 1993). Paul Farmer (1996) has argued that our present conceptual approach to the epidemiology of infectious disease is inappropriate. Our preoccupation with identifying changes in ambient-environmental niches for infectious agents leads us to overlook these more fundamental influences. He argues that the so-called 're-emergence' of tuberculosis in the USA, entails a recent uncovering of a disease that has long been present in the poor. That view also implies that the high rates of tuberculosis in immigrants to the USA reflect general characteristics of the country of their origin, rather than the circumstances of poverty, inequality and warfare that typically lead to emigration (Truong *et al*, 1997).

As with tuberculosis, HIV infection is now entrenching itself among the world's poor and disempowered, especially in sub-Saharan Africa and South Asia. Contrary to conventional descriptions of the inter-continental spread of HIV, Farmer (1996) argues that 'much of the spread of HIV in the 1970s and 1980s moved along international "fault lines" tracking along steep gradients of inequality, which are also paths of migrant labour and sexual commerce'. He suggests that our research models should be based more on fluid biosocial networks through which microbes move rather than on routine surveillance in relation to fixed political-administrative units.

How might the changes in agricultural practice associated with the emergence of Argentine and Bolivian viral haemorrhagic fever (see above) have been related to international trade agreements? Consider the example, from early 1997, of hepatitis A imported into the USA in strawberries from Mexico. This incident appears to reflect the dark underside of free trade agreements. In negotiating the North American Free Trade Agreement, human welfare issues such as the provision of good wages and toilet facilities to workers, and enforcement of environmental standards, were minimized; the notion that Latino farm-workers should be treated and paid well was considered a profit-endangering cost. The subsequent faecal contamination of imported strawberries from Mexico is not, therefore, surprising.

The ideology of deregulated market-forces, with its resultant socioeconomic inequalities, is in the ascendant in today's world. Yet, by perpetuating poverty, destabilising environments and communities, and increasing the rich—poor divide, it contributes significantly to many of the world's persisting and emerging infectious diseases. Under the fashionable banner of competition, market efficiency, profitability and comparative advantage, the tempo and scale of economic globalization have proceeded faster than ever in the 1990s, even as its corrosive social, cultural and environmental impacts have become more evident.

Economic disincentives and the international pharmaceutical industry

In today's market-driven global economy, national governments have increasingly withdrawn to the sidelines, and the impulse for rich nations to assist poor nations is waning. One symptom of this trend is the approximately 100-fold difference in per person expenditure on pharmaceuticals between rich and poor nations. In this setting, the commercial priorities of the private sector in today's world of increasingly deregulated and globalised capital can directly affect public health risks.

Consider the increasing problem of sleeping sickness (trypanosomiasis) in Africa. There are today an estimated 250 000–300 000 cases of sleeping sickness scattered through thousands of villages in central Africa. The disease is caused by trypanosomes that infect the blood, lymph nodes, and eventually the brain. Trypanosomiasis occurs naturally in the herds of native ungulates of eastern Africa, with little effect on health. However, the disease vector, the tsetse fly, also feeds on the blood of humans and their cattle.

In earlier centuries, this disease was probably widespread in much of Africa. The European colonial regimes in Africa introduced highly successful campaigns to control the disease, and almost eradicated it. However, since the era of national independence in the 1960s these control measures have been allowed to lapse in many African countries. This decade, the estimated annual incidence of sleeping sickness has risen approximately ten-fold—especially in strife-riven central African countries.

While the untreated disease is nearly always fatal, among patients treated early the cure rate exceeds 90%. However, continuing production of the arsenic-containing drug Melarsoprol used most frequently to treat advanced cases of sleeping sickness is in jeopardy as production of the drug is technically difficult and, without subsidy, it is unprofitable. Furthermore, environmentalists in Germany have been seeking a ban on the production of the arsenical molecule because the toxic byproducts contaminate rivers and subterranean waters. Here, again, the corrosive combination of market forces and politics intervenes as the rich world becomes less willing to invest on behalf of the health of poor populations.

Conclusions

Our world accommodates a restless parasitism in which the human species has always been just one of the players. As human ecology changes, so do patterns of infectious diseases. We are inextricably bound up with the natural world, a world of competition and symbiosis between organisms great and small. Thus patterns of infectious disease have changed as human populations have moved from nomadism to agrarianism to industrial urbanization.

We are currently living through a major transition in human ecology. This transition, like its predecessors, has great consequences for the profile of infectious diseases. The first such transition undertaken by the modern human species, the diaspora out of Africa around 100 000 BP, radically altered the epidemiological environment for hunter-gatherers and entailed a large general reduction in exposure to infectious agents. An ice-age later, 10 000 years ago, the agricultural and livestock revolution created extensive new opportunities for microbes. In recent centuries, industrialization, urbanization, and Western social modernization has—especially in the past few decades—opened up auspicious new opportunities for microbes. It has also confronted them with the intense selective pressure of the widespread use of antibiotics.

Today, as the scale of human ecological impact becomes increasingly global, so the probabilities of new and resurgent infectious diseases continue to multiply. Plus ça change.

References

Akhtar R, McMichael AJ. Rainfall and malaria outbreaks in western Rajasthan. *Lancet*, 1996; **348**: 1457–1458

Barthold SW. Globalisation of Lyme borreliosis. *Lancet*, 1996; **348**: 1603–1604

Bouma MJ, van der Kaay HJ. Epidemic malaria in India's Thar desert. *Lancet*, 1995; **346**: 1232–1233

Bouma MJ, van der Kaay HJ. The El Niño Southern Oscillation and the historic malaria epidemics on the Indian subcontinent and Sri Lanka: an early warning system for future epidemics? *Tropical Medicine and International Health*, 1996; **1**: 86–96

Bouma MJ, Sondorp HE, van der Kaay HJ. Climate change and periodic epidemic malaria. *Lancet*, 1994; **343**: 1440

Castilla RE, Sawyer DO. Malaria rates and fate: a socioeconomic study of malaria in Brazil. *Social Science and Medicine*, 1993; **37**: 1137–1145

Colwell RR. Global climate and infectious disease: the cholera paradigm. *Science*, 1996; **274**: 2025–2031

Cook GC. The Asiatic cholera: an historical determinant of human genomic and social structure. In: Drasar BS, Forrest BD (eds), *Cholera and the Ecology of Vibrio cholerae*. London: Chapman & Hall, 1996, pp 18–53

Duchin JS, Koster FT, Peters CJ *et al.* Hantavirus pulmonary syndrome: a clinical description of 17 patients with a newly recognized disease. The Hantavirus Study Group. *New England Journal of Medicine*, 1994; **330**: 949–955

Epstein PR. Detecting climate change: biological and physical signs appear in montane regions. In: Jackson E, Woollard K (eds), *Climate Change and Human Health in the Asia-Pacific*. Amsterdam: Greenpeace International, 1997, pp 25–28

Farmer P. Social inequalities and emerging infectious diseases. *Emerging Infectious Diseases*, 1996; **2**: 258–269

Gubler DJ, Clark GG. Dengue/dengue hemorrhagic fever: the emergence of a global health problem. *Emerging Infectious Diseases*, 1995; **1**: 55–57

Hales S, Weinstein P, Woodward A. Dengue fever epidemics in the South Pacific: driven by El Niño Southern Oscillation? *Lancet*, 1996; **348**: 1664–1665

Harb M, Faris R, Gad AM, Hafez ON, Ramzy R, Buck AA. The resurgence of lymphatic filariasis on the Nile Delta. *Bulletin of the World Health Organization*, 1993; **71:** 49–54

Herrera-Basto E, Prevots DR, Zarate ML, Silva JL, Sepulveda-Amor J. First reported outbreak of classical dengue fever at 1,700 meters above sea level in Guerrero State, Mexico, June 1988. *American Journal of Tropical Medicine and Hygiene*, 1992; **46**: 649–653

Huq A, Colwell RR, Chowdhury MA *et al.* Coexistence of *Vibrio cholerae* 01 and 0139 Bengal in plankton in Bangladesh. *Lancet*, 1995; **345**: 1249

Intergovernmental Panel on Climate Change (IPCC). *Climate Change*, 1995 — *The Science of Climate Change: Contribution of Working Group I to the Second Assessment Report of the Intergovernmental Panel on Climate Change.* Houghton JT, Meira Filho LG, Callander BA *et al* (eds). New York: Cambridge University Press, 1996

Islam MS, Miah MA, Hasan MK, Sack RB, Albert MJ. Detection of non-culturable *Vibrio cholerae* 01 associated with a cyanobacterium from an aquatic environment in Bangladesh. *Transactions of the Royal Society of Tropical Medicine and Hygiene*, 1994; **88**: 298–299

Karlen A. *Plague's Progress: A Social History of Disease.* London: Gollancz, 1995

Last JM. Global change: ozone depletion, greenhouse warming and public health. *Annual Review of Public Health*, 1993; **14**: 115–136

Lifson AR. Mosquitoes, models and dengue. *Lancet*, 1996; **347**: 1201–1202

Martens WJM. *Health Impacts of Climate Change and Ozone Depletion. An Eco-Epidemiological Modelling Approach.* ISBN 90-901405-4. Maastricht, Holland: University of Maastricht, 1997

Martens WJM, Niessen LW, Rotmans J, Jetten TH, McMichael AJ. Potential impact of global climate change on malaria risk. *Environmental Health Perspectives*, 1995; **103**: 458–464

Martin P, Lefebvre M. Malaria and climate: sensitivity of malaria potential transmission to climate. *Ambio*, 1995; **24**: 200–207

Mathieu LG, Sonea S. A powerful bacterial world. *Endeavour*, 1995: 112–117

McNeill WH. *Plagues and Peoples.* New York: Anchor Press, 1976

McNeill WH. Disease emergence in history. In: Morse SS (ed), *Emerging Viruses.* Oxford: Oxford University Press, 1993, pp 29–36

McMichael AJ. *Planetary Overload. Global Environmental Change and the Health of the Human Species.* Cambridge: Cambridge University Press, 1993a

McMichael AJ. Global environmental change and human population health: a conceptual and scientific challenge for epidemiology. *International Journal of Epidemiology*, 1993b; **22**: 1–8

McMichael AJ, Haines A, Slooff R, Kovats S (eds), *Climate Change and Human Health.* WHO/WHG/96.7. Geneva: World Health Organization, 1996

McMichael AJ. Integrated assessment of potential health impacts of global environmental change: prospects and limitations. *Environmental Modelling and Assessment*, 1997; **2**: 129–137

Morse SS. Examining the origins of emerging viruses. In: Morse SS (ed), *Emerging Viruses.* Oxford: Oxford University Press, 1993, pp 10–28

Patz JA, Epstein PR, Burke TA, Balbus JM. Global climate change and emerging infectious diseases. *Journal of the American Medical Association*, 1996; **275**: 217–223

Sawyer D. Economic and social consequences of malaria in new colonization projects in Brazil. *Social Science and Medicine*, 1993; **37**: 1131–1136

Tamplin ML, Carrillo-Parodi C. Environmental spread of *Vibrio cholerae* in Peru. *Lancet*, 1991; **338**: 1216–1217

Thwaites G, Taviner M, Gant V. The English sweating sickness, 1485 to 1551. *New England Journal of Medicine*, 1997; **336**: 580–582

Truong DH, Hedemark LL, Mickman JK, Mosher LB, Dietrich SE, Lowry PW. Tuberculosis among Tibetan immigrants from India and Nepal in Minnesota, 1992–1995. *Journal of the American Medical Association*, 1997; **277**: 735–738

Wilson ME. Infectious disease: an ecological perspective. *British Medical Journal*, 1995; **311**: 1681–1684

3
Emerging diseases and global change: past, present and possible futures

Paul R. Epstein

Center for Health and the Global Environment, Harvard Medical School, Boston, USA

Introduction

Pandemics of infectious disease have occurred in waves that often parallel social transitions and accompanying environmental change. A major characteristic of these periods is the exhaustion of resources and generation of unmanageable wastes, allowing opportunistic species—insects, rodents and micro-organisms—to achieve dominance. Some pandemics have led to the dissolution of the prevailing order; occasionally they have helped propel social action that has reformed the conditions that have caused them.

Today, widespread loss of biodiversity is being compounded by climate change and instability, altering conditions for growth, permissible ranges, environmental selection pressures and host susceptibilities. As we enter a period of environmental stress, we must ask if the symptoms and the potential consequences and costs of this process will be recognized. Given the non-linear behaviour of complex systems, will our consciousness regarding the driving forces be transformed more swiftly than are systems themselves?

Environmental distress syndrome

Ecologists have defined a generalized environmental distress syndrome. The symptoms of this include:

New and Resurgent Infections: Prediction, Detection and Management of Tomorrow's Epidemics.
Edited by B. Greenwood and K. De Cock.

- Emerging infectious diseases (EIDs)
- An overall decline in genetic and species biodiversity
- The growing dominance of 'generalists' such as crows, Canadian geese and gulls that have wide-ranging diets over 'specialists' (like plovers) which occupy localized niches that are disappearing
- The decline in one type of specialist—the pollinators (bees, birds, bats, butterflies and beetles)—whose niches and activities fit with, and are indispensable for, the preservation of flowering plants
- The proliferation of harmful algal blooms along coastlines.

Regulatory mechanisms

A major symptom of a generalized environmental distress syndrome is the emergence of new diseases, resurgence of old diseases and redistribution of vector-borne diseases on a global scale. The World Health Organization reports that 30 new diseases have emerged in the past two decades.

Are we reaching limits to natural systems that regulate pests? Mechanisms that regulate harmful mutations and species invasions at the level of individual organisms are mirrored by interspecific actions existing at a more general level which prevent opportunistic species from overexploiting and dominating all but the most degraded of natural systems. Weeds, rodents, insects and micro-organisms are opportunists, excelling at 'r-selected' attributes; that is, they reproduce rapidly, have huge broods, small body sizes, wide-ranging appetites and are good at dispersal and colonization of new environments. In stable environments, large predators fare well and keep opportunistic species under control.

The relative balance between functional groups (e.g. predators and prey, scavengers and decomposers) maintains the resilience and resistance of ecosystems and helps keep opportunistic organisms from overgrowing environments. But in degraded environments, opportunists can seize the upper hand, just as opportunistic infections (OIs) can take advantage of patients with weakened immune systems.

Predator/prey relationships are central to biological control. Owls, coyotes and snakes help regulate populations of rodents—opportunistic species involved in the transmission of Lyme disease, hantaviruses, arenaviruses, leptospirosis and human plague. Freshwater fish, reptiles and bats help limit the abundance of mosquitoes, some of which carry malaria, yellow fever, dengue fever and many encephalitides. Finfish, shellfish and sea mammals affect the dynamics of coastal algal populations. Some algae are toxic ('red tides'), while others ('brown tides') cause hypoxia, harming seagrasses and shellfish beds. Still others can harbour pathogens like *Vibrio cholerae*, and other Gram-negative bacteria (Byrd *et al*, 1991; Epstein, 1992a). The discovery of a coastal reservoir for *V. cholerae* may be just the 'tip of the iceberg' as far as marine and estuarine sources of seafood- and recreation-related illness are concerned. Rodents, insects and algae represent key biological indicators, which respond rapidly to environmental change. The current rate of extinctions assumes additional significance in this respect. Periods of mass extinctions—punctuations in evolutionary equilibrium—are followed by the emergence of new species. Will such a collapse initially favour opportunistic species?

Synergies

Rodents are a growing problem in the USA, Latin America, Africa, Europe, Asia and Australia. Rodents—pre-eminent opportunists—are believed to be the fastest reproducing mammal. They eat everything humans do, thrive on contaminated water and food, and are even great swimmers. Rodents consume 20% of the world's growing and stored grain, 13% in the USA, and up to 75% in some African nations. Rodents also carry diseases.

Several environmental factors can act synergistically to precipitate explosions of nuisance organisms. In Bolivia, for example, the rodent-borne Machupo virus emerged in 1962 when land-clearing shifted species dominance from forest to field mice (Calomys) and when excessive use of pesticides killed off predators. Bolivian haemorrhagic fever, which had killed 10–20% of the small local population, subsided when cats were reintroduced. Similar synergies gave rise to Junin virus infections in Argentina, Guaranito in Venezuela and Sabia in Brazil.

Variations in climate can also destabilize natural biological controls. In the south-west USA, prolonged drought (1987–92) reduced mouse predators (owls, snakes, coyotes) while heavy rains in 1993 supplied food (grasshoppers and pinon nuts) and led to a 10-fold explosion of *Peromyscus maniculatus*—a rodent associated with the emergence of Hantavirus Pulmonary Syndrome. An experiment with Canadian rabbits is illustrative of the importance of synergy. Removal of predators doubles populations; food supplements triple them; together, an 11-fold explosion in population occurs (Stenseth, 1995; Krebs *et al*, 1995).

In southern Africa, rodent populations exploded in 1994 following the 1993 and 1994 rains that succeeded a prolonged drought during the preceding six years. Avian and land predators were virtually absent, and draught animals had succumbed, leaving underground rodent burrows intact. The maize crop in Zimbabwe was crippled and, soon after, human plague broke out in Zimbabwe and on the borders of neighbouring Malawi and Mozambique. Subsequently, a rodent-borne virus killed 81 elephants in South Africa's Kruger Park, threatening tourism.

Rodent-borne hantaviruses have resurged in several European nations, particularly in former Yugoslavia, and rodent-borne diseases like leptospirosis are reported increasingly in urban centres in the USA, where sanitation has declined. In late 1996, hantavirus infection emerged in western Argentina where at least 10 deaths have frightened off tourists and threaten the livelihood of the region.

In India, plague resurged in 1994, following a blistering summer (124°F, or 51°C), which had left animals prostrate across the north and created furnaces for fleas in houses with stored grains. The unusually heavy monsoons following the heatwave led to population crowding in Surat and an apparent outbreak of pneumonic (person-to-person) plague. Upsurges in malaria and dengue fever also followed the flooding. Finally, in Australia in 1995, rodents emerged as crop pests following five years of drought that was associated with the prolonged El Niño activity of the first half of this decade.

Current land-use practices, overuse of chemicals to control pests and increased climate variability may increase the chances for 'nasty synergies'. Habitat loss and climate change may act synergistically, the former preventing species migration in response to the latter. A disturbance in one factor can be destabilising; multiple perturbations can affect the resistance and the resilience of a system.

Pathogen evolution

There are many selection pressures that affect the evolution of pathogens. One that is often ignored is host nutrition. Evidence that malnutrition and depressed immune surveillance systems may allow evolution of virulence at rates beyond baseline comes from an experiment with mice and coxsackie viruses that cause cardiac disease in China (Beck *et al*, 1995). In mice deprived of selenium, benign coxsackie viruses mutate more rapidly than baseline to become pathogens. Transferred to healthy mice, they cause disease. The implication of this experiment is that what happens in poor, malnourished populations can affect the wealthier and healthier communities and nations.

Did such factors play a role in the emergence of HIV? Did years of malnutrition in Africa (from land degradation and export-driven monocropping) combined with an increasing burden of disease weaken immune surveillance systems (Epstein and Packard, 1987)? Just as new OIs develop in those with HIV/AIDS, did a previously benign, slow-growing virus evolve to become a pathogen in the face of inadequate defence systems?

Stressful conditions may encourage mutations. While the notion of 'directed evolution'—mutations directed by environmental conditions—is difficult to believe, it is possible, and eminently plausible, that a hypermutability state is induced in response to various types of stresses (Lamarck meets Darwin?) (Beardsley, 1997).

Toxins can cause mutations in structural and also in regulatory genes, thus destabilising internal controls over mutations. Toxins can also act at the ecosystem level, altering the balance of species that preserve ecosystem function and structure. Predators and pollinators are disproportionately affected by toxins, their prey reproducing rapidly, evolving (resistance) and rebounding with punishing ferocity as Carson (1962) eloquently depicted—absent in a Silent

Spring. An ecological risk assessment of chemicals (and other human activities) must include their impact on species' abundance and composition. Antibiotics represent another important group of chemicals that when used extensively in agricultural practices as well as human medicine can lead to the emergence of resistant pathogens (see Levin, this volume, chapter 5).

Recently another type of agent has emerged—the prion. This destabilized cell surface protein that spreads its influence in a cascading, infectious manner may have originated from mutations or from directly damaged proteins. Have environmental elements played a role in its appearance? Are organophosphates and other toxins playing a contributory role in destabilizing cell surface proteins, or the genes that generate them? A potential link between chemical contamination of our environment and infectious diseases deserves further exploration.

Pandemics in history

Is the current global resurgence of infectious disease a new phenomenon? From a long-term historical perspective, pandemics have often been associated with major historical transitions and they have had profound impacts on human development.

A pandemic occurred as the Roman Empire declined (AD 541, Plague of Justinian) (organism disputed) and raged for two centuries, claiming over 40 million lives. Urban centres in Europe were abandoned and populations resettled into rural, feudal communities.

After a 600-year hiatus, plague (due to *Yersinia pestis*) reappeared in the Middle Ages (AD 1346), when urban populations had once again outstripped their infrastructure. There were several compounding factors. Human populations had migrated from East to West, the Medieval Warm Period may have contributed to a proliferation of rats and fleas, and cats had been killed in the belief that they were witches. In the ensuing five years, plague killed 25 million people, or 30% of Europe's population.

Development in Europe from the mid-18th to the first third of the 19th century was accompanied by a sharp decline in infectious disease mortality. However, from 1790 to 1850 European cities grew seven-fold and as a result became breeding grounds for three major infectious diseases—cholera, smallpox and tuberculosis. This resurgence of infectious disease helped to precipitate protests throughout Europe, and ultimately led to constructive responses. In the UK, the Sanitary and Environmental Reform Movements began and the development of epidemiology ushered in modern public health principles, setting the stage for a national health programme (Epstein, 1992b).

Recent history

By the 1960s, improvements in hygiene, sanitation and mosquito control led most public health authorities to believe that humans would prevail over infectious diseases. Public health schools turned their attention to chronic ailments, and the environmental underpinning needed for the control of infectious diseases was all but abandoned as a field of instruction. With the resurgence of infectious diseases in the 1980s, the ground has shifted dramatically.

According to *The World Health Report 1996* (WHO, 1996) 'drug-resistant strains of bacteria and other microbes are having a deadly impact on the fight against tuberculosis, malaria, cholera, diarrhea and pneumonia—which collectively killed more than 10 million people in 1995'. Vaccine-preventable diseases have reappeared. The incidence of diphtheria has risen exponentially in the former USSR (4000 cases in 1992, 8000 in 1993 and 48 000 in 1994), and the disease has spread to 15 Eastern European countries, although by 1995 its incidence had levelled off following the implementation of immunization programmes.

Malaria, infecting half a billion persons yearly and killing one to three million annually, is resurgent and growing evermore resistant to drugs. In the present decade the worldwide incidence of this infection has quadrupled. Dengue fever, which had virtually disappeared from the Americas by the 1970s, has resurged in that continent and infected over 240 000 people in 1995. In 1996, over 8000 cases of dengue and several hundred deaths were recorded in New Delhi. Peri-urban settlements and proliferation of non-biodegradable containers provide mosquito breeder sites. In 1995 the largest epidemic of yellow fever since 1950 occurred in the Americas; Peru and the Amazon basin were heavily affected.

In 1966 the largest ever recorded epidemic of meningitis, associated with drought in Africa, struck West Africa. Over 100 000 persons contracted the disease and over 10 000 died. Conditions conducive to emerging infectious diseases are now worldwide, according to a WHO report (WHO, 1996). Diseases like Hantavirus Pulmonary Syndrome and Lyme disease are not imported diseases into the US; the conditions for their spread are present in the US itself, just as the conditions for the spread of tuberculosis are present in shelters for the homeless and in prisons. In 1995, US mortality rates from infectious diseases increased 58% (Pinner *et al*, 1996).

While some of the time periods discussed above are extensive, others are short, and we can ask if we have entered a historical period of accelerated change in social, ecological and climatic conditions. If so, what are the biological indicators? Will we perceive the symptoms of these changes and take corrective measures before we exceed the resilience of the system?

Climate change and vector-borne diseases

Insects and insect-borne diseases are currently being reported at higher altitudes than previously in Africa, Asia and Latin America. Highland malaria (particularly falciparum malaria, perhaps the most temperature-sensitive form) is becoming a problem for rural highland regions of Papua New Guinea (Rozendaal, 1996), for highlands in the Americas (Koopman *et al*, 1991), and may soon threaten urban centres in Central Africa. In 1995, dengue fever blanketed the Americas, crossing mountain ranges that had previously presented barriers to spread (data from the Pan American Health Organization, 1996). Upward migration of plants has been documented on 30 Alpine peaks (Grabherr *et al*, 1994; Pauli *et al*, 1996) and has been observed in Alaska, the US Sierra Nevada and New Zealand (Yoon, 1994). Moreover, these biological findings are occurring in tandem with widespread physical changes. Montane glaciers are in retreat in Argentina, Peru, Alaska, Iceland, Norway, the Swiss Alps, Kenya, the Himalayas, Indonesia and New Zealand (Kaser and Noggler, 1991; Hastenrath and Kruss, 1992; Thompson *et al*, 1993; Haeberli, 1995; IPCC, 1996).

Temperature measurements provide direct evidence of climatic changes. Using radiosonde measurements, Diaz and Graham (1996) have reported a 160 metre rise in the freezing level in the mountains since 1970 (about 1°C, based on the adiabatic lapse rate).

Recent models and data that combine the effects of greenhouse gases with stratospheric ozone depletion and aerosolized sulfates predict the most warming in the mid-troposphere of the Southern Hemisphere, surpassing the warming evident on the Earth's surface.

Ocean warming

Deep ocean warming has been reported along subtropical transects in the tropical Pacific, Atlantic and Indian Oceans, at both poles and in the Arctic tundra. Water evaporating from warmer seas increases the hydrological cycle, reinforcing the greenhouse effect, and warm seas can fuel hurricane intensity. Ocean warming may be harming marine plankton and warming has been associated with a shift in marine flora and fauna along the California coast since the 1930s (Barry *et al*, 1995).

Harmful algal blooms of increasing extent, duration and intensity, and involving new species, are being reported from nations throughout the globe. Indeed, 'the worldwide increase in coastal algal blooms may be one of the first biological signs of global change' (T. Smayda, personal communication, 1995).

The growth of coastal algae is stimulated by excess nutrients (sewage, fertilizers and aerosolized nitrogen), destruction of wetlands (filters of nutrients) and overfishing (reducing predation). Warming and stratification of the water column can also contribute to the proliferation of coastal algal blooms by increasing photosynthesis, metabolism and by shifting species composition to more toxic cyanobacteria and dinoflagellates. The increased incidence, intensity, duration, and appearance of novel toxic species of harmful algal blooms (HABs), may be one of the first biological signs of global change. One can visualize this phenomenon with the aid of remotely sensed satellite images.

The 1990s

From 1990 to 1995 the Pacific persisted in the warm El Niño/Southern Oscillation (ENSO) phase. Since 1877 no El Niño has endured for more than three years; and both anomalous phases bring climatic extremes to many regions across the globe. Accompanying the subsequent cold phase (La Niña) of 1995/96, many regions of the globe that had experienced drought experienced intense rains and flooding. As in Colombia, floods in Southern Africa were accompanied by an upsurge of vector-borne diseases such as malaria. Other areas experienced the reverse, with drought and fires replacing floods. During 1996 world grain stores fell to their lowest level since the 1930s.

Weather is always variable, but increased variability and rapid temperature fluctuations associated with a less stable jet stream may be characteristic of our changing climate system. Increased variability and weather volatility can have significant consequences for health and for society.

Decadal variability

The cumulative ecological impacts of the prolonged El Niño (5 years and 8 months) have yet to be evaluated. Consider the following biological events. In 1995, warming in the Caribbean led to coral bleaching for the first time in Belize, as sea-surface temperatures surpassed the 29°C threshold. The warm Caribbean provided moisture for the north-east storms of 1995/96, and continues to do so into 1997. The La Niña in the eastern Pacific altered the jet stream, providing condensing cold conditions in areas opposite to those affected during the previous El Niño. Insects proliferated in New Orleans, there was another widespread die-off of Caribbean sea urchins (1995), and a die-off of manatees and shore birds following a *Gymnodium breve* red tide along Florida's coast (1996). These events could be examples of the cumulative impacts of the 'longest [El Niño period] on record' (Trenberth and Hoar, 1996).

Did prolonged El Niño conditions, a warmed Caribbean and a warmed Gulf Stream contribute to the current warming of the Northern Atlantic, altering the North Atlantic Oscillation (NAO) and shifting the Atlantic dipole?

Gray (Colorado State University) has recalculated his formula for predicting hurricanes based on the change in Atlantic sea-surface temperatures (SSTs), stating that conditions appear to have reverted to those of the 1930s and 1940s when hurricane activity was more intense (Cowen, 1997). A new twist arrived in the spring of 1997, with warming SSTs in the Pacific ushering in the largest El Niño of the century. El Niño changes the jet stream and trade winds, keeping storms off the US eastern seaboard. However, the combined changes in the Atlantic and the Pacific (ENSO and the NAO being two modes in which climate dynamics express themselves), may have contributed to the massive flooding in central Europe (especially Poland and Germany) that occurred in July 1997.

Increasing ocean temperatures are associated with the isotherm shift described

(Diaz and Graham, 1996), and the world's oceans may indeed be the main repository (capacitor) for the past century's global warming. More basin-wide data are needed to evaluate the trends currently detected.

Greenland ice cores and Atlantic plankton fossils are consistent in depicting rapid climate change (RCC) events over the period of a few years, coincident with changes in ocean circulation and the 'great conveyor belt'. According to plankton records, the next Heinrich event—calving of the polar ice caps—is due in AD 3200, as determined by precessional (Malenkovitch) cycles, when the Earth's axis brings its northern hemisphere closest to the Sun in summer (perihelion).

Costs of extreme weather events and epidemics

Irrespective of the origins of climate instability, the rise in severe wind- and flood-related events worldwide has had extraordinary consequences for property insurers. In the USA, prior to 1989, no single event had ever led to losses exceeding US$1 billion. Since then, annual losses have risen dramatically—from US$1.6 billion annually in the 1980s to US$12 billion annually in the 1990s (only partially explained by increased 'exposure'). In the USA the main causes of losses to insurers include: Hurricane Hugo, 1989—US$5.4 billion; Hurricane Andrew, 1992–US$16.5 billion; the winter storms of 1993—US$1.8 billion; the 1993 summer floods—US$10 billion; and, most recently, Hurricane Opal, 1995—US$2.1 billion; 1996 blizzard, drought, fires, tornadoes—as yet untallied; 1997 floods and ice storms—human and property casualties climbing.

The Munich Reinsurance year-end review concluded that 600 disasters in 1996 cost the industry US$60 billion. Increased exposure was compounded by new extremes of temperature, rainfall and wind. Storms and floods accounted for more than half of the disasters (Fisher, 1996).

The costs to the insurance industry are perhaps the best indication of the non-sustainability of current practices. With continuing extreme climatic variability, health and environmental costs may grow. The American Academy of Actuaries and Standard & Poor's already estimate that health-related and environmental restoration claims over the next 30 years may reach US$50–125 billion, leaving a reserve shortfall equal to about one-third of the insurance industry's capital. Actuarial calculations must also take into account non-linearities and 'jumps' in system states.

The impacts of disease of humans, agriculture and livestock can also be costly. While the 1991 cholera epidemic cost Peru over US$1 billion, airline and hotel industries lost from US$2 to US$5 billion from the 1994 Indian plague. Cruise boats are turning away from Caribbean islands racked by dengue fever, threatening that region's US$12 billion tourist industry (employing over 500 000 people). The global resurgence of malaria, dengue fever and cholera, and emergence of relatively new diseases like Ebola, toxic *Escherichia coli* and bovine spongiform encephalitis (BSE), can affect eating habits, trade, tourism and politics.

What may the future hold?

As we approach the next century, we can expect the spread of infectious diseases. Vector-borne diseases continue to appear at higher altitudes and latitudes, and persist longer during the year in areas where they now exist, in agreement with model projections. Antibiotic-resistant organisms will undoubtedly continue to appear, causing increasing problems for health-care institutions despite recent breakthroughs in gene therapy aimed at restoring antibiotic sensitivity. There will be new surprises, and the emergence of new viral, bacterial and protozoan illnesses.

Water safety and supply, quality and quantity, will undoubtedly become critical. Water quality is threatened by the persistent flow of industrial wastes, sewage, fertilisers, aerosolised nitrogen and farm run-off. Compounded by extreme weather events that increase effluents of chemicals and micro-organisms, contamination of water supplies, particularly with protozoa that are insensitive to chlorine, will most likely increase. Agriculture now takes up over 85% of water supplies, and our impoundments and uses of rivers have altered local hydrology. In some areas, rivers that once flowed into oceans no longer reach them. Conflicts over river ways are bound to become more acute, just as are conflicts over dwindling fisheries.

Given the current rise in food-borne illness and poor agricultural growing conditions, we may project a continuing threat from food-borne illness in the future. Irradicating food at the borders of developed nations—one manifestation of the evolving fortress mentality in the face of emerging global issues—is not foolproof and the practice puts off addressing the underlying socio-economic conditions. Shellfish and finfish contamination is increasing in frequency, and one may expect continued coastal pollution and warming to exacerbate this trend. The contamination of meat with toxic *E. coli* in Scotland, Japan and the USA, and the emergence of other gastroenteric pathogens and prions, magnify the ecological issues raised by extensive land clearing and cattle raising. This and the threat to fisheries by disease and overfishing will call into question our dietary dependency upon animal protein in the coming century.

While surveillance methods for water and food safety may improve, efforts to address prevention are in their infancy. Such measures would include changing farming practices, maintaining upstream riparian (river-edge) wetlands that filter waste, and improving techniques for food preparation.

The forecast for the near future may not appear bright. Increasing fragmentation and intoxification of habitats will continue to harm predators and other key elements of environmental regulatory relationships. There is strong evidence that warming above and below us will continue, with great instability in weather patterns being its manifestation on the Earth's surface.

Many questions remain. Is the Earth's surface relatively protected from the warming by sulfate-enhanced clouds? Are the changing weather patterns reflective of changing ocean heat retention and irregular release? There are as yet poorly understood feedback mechanisms that have kept ocean salinity, atmospheric oxygen and average global temperatures relatively stable for thousands of years. Do the extremes reflect overshoots in these dynamical feedback systems? For example, the La Niña—cooling of the eastern Pacific—that followed the longest El Niño on record (1990–95), delivered rains to regions that had been parched for much of the preceding five years.

These ENSO conditions alter the jet stream and affect weather patterns worldwide. In the 1990s, the jet stream is behaving differently than it did in previous decades. Are the heat, chemical and hydrological fluxes within the system—from land, atmosphere, oceans and cryosphere—changing, and at what rate? If spring is coming early, and oceans are the chief repository for global warming, are we approaching such an event sooner than projected? When does the accumulation of strange and destabilising attractors coalesce to destabilize the central attractor of the climate system?

Under the increasing burden of debt, unequal terms of trade and structural adjustment programmes, the regulatory functions of many nation-states are being eroded. This pattern is most evident in Africa, but there are similar pressures in Latin America from Mexico to Argentina, and in central and south-east Asia. The dissolution of states in Africa and parts of Europe damages economies and the environment, and has led to devastating wars of clashing ethnic groups. The consequences of war for public health (Levy and Sidel, 1997) could be enormous. In the Balkans, for example, hantaviruses have emerged along with the continued plague of landmines and disrupted infrastructure. In Rwanda, in 1994, the world watched what may be the most intense epidemic of modern times, when 40 000 deaths occurred over a period of weeks from cholera.

On the other hand, if our present course is truly non-sustainable, this will be manifest in economic terms. The threats to the financial sector, first evident in the US$1.4 trillion property insurance industry, may present international industry with a critical dilemma. Ultimately, using resources efficiently and generating energy with renewable sources will become economically as well as environmentally necessary. When will this happen?

Conclusions

Extreme weather events are sure to plague nations throughout the world. Infectious diseases, reflective of social inequity and disintegration, altered ecologies, and climate change will continue to appear, affecting humans, livestock, agriculture and marine life.

While some argue that the increases in infectious diseases may limit human population growth, the real fear is that pests and pathogens affecting marine and terrestrial animals, agricultural crops and forest systems will also proliferate. The ‘limits to growth’ will undoubtedly express themselves in the areas of food, water and health, three basic needs. These aspects of emerging infectious diseases threaten food security, biological security and life-support systems themselves.

What can be done to limit the impact of these changes? The health professions have an important role to play. They must unite forces with biologists of all kinds, with atmospheric chemists, social scientists and historians to present an integrated picture of the changes that are occurring and of their consequences. Macroeconomic forces are overriding projects and policies designed to stimulate economic growth while preserving the environment. This de-coupling of microforces, and subsystems, from the goals and directions of the larger systems, lies at the heart of increasing income inequality, mass movements of populations, weakening of nation states and their inability to develop healthy economies.

A new economic and regulatory framework is needed, to stimulate renewables, and to encourage environmental restoration. While the periphery may be privatized, the centre must determine the relationships among the parts. Global regulations and governance over the behaviour of the multinationals are necessary for the preservation of healthy, sustainable economies. Without such acceptance of the need for international governance by the currently unregulated and uncontrolled, the 'tragedy of the commons' (Hardin, 1968), where individuals gain as the collective loses, may lead to the autocratic imposition of order.

In place of the current economic order, there must be positive financial incentives to develop renewables and use resources sustainably. We must begin to switch subsidies from activities destructive to the environment to those that maintain it, and to remove the negative incentives that now drive local activities that are rapidly deteriorating our common environment.

Our task is to understand the global nature of the environmental distress syndrome and to indicate the pathways that provide positive incentives for healthy growth. Ideas and values can also change abruptly. We can only hope that consciousness regarding the finite limits of Earth's resources, and the way we use what is available, will change more rapidly than do the natural systems we all depend upon.

References

Barry JP, Baxter CH, Sagarin RD, Gilman SE. Climate-related, long-term faunal changes in a California rocky intertidal community. *Science*, 1995; **267**: 672–675

Beardsley T. Evolution evolving. *Scientific American*, 1997; **277(3)**:15–18

Beck MA, Shi Q, Morris VC, Levander OA. Rapid genomic evolution of a non-virulent coxsackievirus B3 in selenium-deficient mice results in selection of identical virulent isolates. *Nature Medicine*, 1995; **1**: 433–436

Byrd JJ, Xu HS, Colwell RR. Viable but non-culturable bacteria in drinking water. *Applied Environmental Microbiology*, 1991; **57**: 875–878

Carson R. *Silent Spring*. Boston: Houghton Miflin, 1962

Cowen RC. Science column. *Christian Science Monitor*, 1 July 1997

Diaz HF, Graham NE. Recent changes in tropical freezing heights and the role of sea surface temperature. *Nature*, 1996; **383**: 152–155

Epstein PR. Cholera and the environment. *Lancet*, 1992a; **338**: 1167–1168

Epstein PR. Pestilence and poverty—historical transitions and the great pandemics. *American Journal of Preventive Medicine*, 1992b; **8**: 263–265

Epstein PR, Packard R. Ecology and immunology. The social context of AIDS in Africa. *Science for the People*, 1987; **19**: 110–117

Fisher A. US insurers take a new look at catastrophes. *Financial Times*, 30 December 1996

Grabherr G, Gottfried N, Pauli H. Climate effects on mountain plants. *Nature*, 1994; **369**: 447

Haeberli W. Climate change impacts on glaciers and permafrost. In: Guisan A, Holton JI, Spichiger R, Tessier L (eds), *Potential Ecological Impacts of Climate Change in the Alps and Fennoscandinavian Mountains*. Geneva: Editions Conserv Bot Geneve, 1995, pp 97–103

Hardin G. The tragedy of the commons. The population problem has no technical solution; it requires a fundamental extension in morality. *Science*, 1968; **162**: 1243–1248

Hastenrath S, Kruss PD. Greenhouse indicators in Kenya. *Nature*, 1992; **355**: 503

Intergovernmental Panel on Climate Change (IPCC). Climate Change '95: The Science of Climate Change. Contribution of Working Group 1 to: Houghton JT, Meiro Filho LG, Callandar BA *et al* (eds), The Second Assessment Report of the IPCC. Cambridge: Cambridge University Press, 1996, pp 149, 370–374

Kaser G, Noggler B. Observations on Speke Glacier, Ruwenzori Range, Uganda. *Journal of Glaciology*, 1991; **37**: 313

Koopman JS, Prevots DR, Vaca-Marin MA *et al.* Determinants and predictors of dengue infection in Mexico. *American Journal of Epidemiology*, 1991; **133**: 1168–1178

Krebs CJ, Boutin S, Boonstra R *et al.* Impact of food and predation on the snowshoe hare cycle. *Science*, 1995; **269**: 1112–1115

Levy BS, Sidel VW (eds). *War and Public Health*. New York: Oxford University Press, 1997

Pauli H, Gottfried M, Grabherr G. Effects of climate change on mountain ecosystems—upward shifting of alpine plants. *World Resource Review*, 1996; **8**: 382–390

Pinner RW, Teutsch SM, Simonsen L *et al.* Trends in infectious disease mortality in the United States. *Journal of the American Medical Association*, 1996; **275**: 189–193

Rozendaal J. *Assignment Report: Malaria. World Health Organization. Pt. Moresby. Papua New Guinea*. Geneva: World Health Organization, 1996

Stenseth NC. Snowshoe hare populations squeezed from below and above. *Science*, 1995; **269**: 1061–1062

Thompson LG, Mosley-Thompson E, Davis M *et al.* 'Recent warming': ice core evidence from tropical ice cores with emphasis on Central Asia. *Global and Planetary Change*, 1993; **7**: 145

Trenberth KE, Hoar TJ. The 1990–1995 El Niño–Southern Oscillation event: longest on record. *Geophysical Research Letters*, 1996; **23**: 57–60

World Health Organization. *World Health Report, 1996: Fighting Disease, Fostering Development*. Geneva: World Health Organization, 1996

Yoon CK. Warming moves plants to peaks threatening extinction. *The New York Times*, 21 June 1994: C4

4
Biological variability in viral pathogens

Andrew McMichael

Institute of Molecular Medicine, John Radcliffe Hospital, Oxford, UK

Biological variability in pathogens is well known, and several examples have been studied in considerable detail. This review concentrates on two virus pathogens, influenza virus and human immunodeficiency virus (HIV), and their relationship with the host immune response. Several general lessons can be learned from these viruses, but there are unique features to each.

Influenza

Influenza virus causes an epidemic, self-limiting infection (Askonas *et al*, 1982). Other viruses, with a similar ability to vary, cause similar illnesses, generally known as 'flu; these include respiratory syncytial viruses, rhinoviruses and adenoviruses. Influenza virus was isolated first in 1934 and has been the subject of intense investigation. There are good descriptions of influenza going back for several hundred years (reviewed in Noble, 1982), and it is clear that large-scale pandemics have occurred at irregular intervals during this period. In this century, there was a catastrophic pandemic in 1918–19 and serious pandemics in 1957 and 1968. Pandemic influenza virus infection causes huge numbers of cases worldwide and it seems that pre-existing immunity, resulting from previous influenza infection, is largely ineffective (Askonas *et al*, 1982). Molecular characterization of influenza viruses has revealed the probable reasons why this is the case (Webster *et al*, 1982). New pandemic strains carry new forms of the virus surface glycoproteins, haemagglutinin (H) and neuraminidase (N). These are acquired by reassortment from animal reservoirs, particularly from pigs and ducks; the two most recent pandemics arose in south-east Asia, where farming of pigs and ducks together is common.

Until recently, it was assumed that the 1918 pandemic, which killed over 20 million people, was caused by a swine influenza of the H1N1 type (Noble, 1982).

New and Resurgent Infections: Prediction, Detection and Management of Tomorrow's Epidemics.
Edited by B. Greenwood and K. De Cock.

This has now been proven by PCR amplification of virus from lung sections of an American soldier who died in the United States in 1918 (Taubenberger *et al*, 1997). The virus obtained from this sample was of the H1N1 type and in phylogenetic trees of nucleotide sequences maps at the root of the tree close to swine H1N1 virus types. Evolution of this virus has been followed in detail. H1N1 viruses predominated until 1957, when they were replaced by the sudden emergence of Asian influenza, H2N2. However, H1N1 viruses returned in 1977, infecting individuals under the age of about 22 years, and this virus has persisted since then, although its prevalence appears to be declining. The protection against H1N1 observed in older age groups in 1977 and subsequently is remarkable and is very probably due to residual immunological memory and resulting protective antibody (Glass *et al*, 1978). The appearance of H2N2 virus in 1957 was associated with a serious pandemic with many deaths. This virus circulated until 1968 when it was replaced by Hong Kong influenza, H3N2, which again caused a pandemic with many deaths. H3N2 virus has persisted since 1968 and has been the major cause of influenza epidemics in recent years. Each new pandemic virus evolves in succeeding years by antigenic drift and selection by the neutralizing humoral immune response of the population as a whole (Wiley *et al*, 1981; Gojobori *et al*, 1994). The surface of each virus evolves dramatically over the years, and H3N2 viruses have changed considerably since their first appearance. In 1997 a new virus, H5N1, appeared in Hong Kong, causing concern about a possible new pandemic (Claas *et al*, 1998).

The immune response to influenza virus is largely cellular during the acute infection (Yap and Ada, 1978). Neutralizing antibody appears first after the bulk of the virus has been eliminated (Yap and Ada, 1978) but is very efficient at protecting against reinfection with the same virus (Webster *et al*, 1982). Vaccines are based on current and predicted circulating viruses and are aimed at generating neutralizing antibodies. The internal proteins of the virus, which stimulate the cellular immune responses, particularly cytotoxic T-lymphocyte responses (CTL), change much more slowly and there is little or no evidence for immune selection. CTL are largely responsible for clearing viraemia in the acute phase of the infection, destroying virus-infected cells before they produce new virus (Yap and Ada, 1978) and releasing interferon-gamma (Morris *et al*, 1982). T-helper cells can also contribute, and mice manipulated so that they have no classical CTL are able to clear virus, though less efficiently than normal mice (Lightman *et al*, 1987).

There is no real evidence that the genetic make-up of human populations has had any major influence on the selection of influenza virus variants. However, influenza virus infection may have had strong selective effects on the genetics of human populations. Whereas all normal humans can make good antibody responses to influenza virus, cellular immune responses vary in specificity according to the HLA- or tissue-type of the infected person (McMichael *et al*, 1986). CTL recognise small peptide fragments of viral proteins that are bound to HLA class I molecules on the surface of infected cells (Townsend *et al*, 1986;

Bjorkman *et al*, 1987). Different HLA types bind and present different peptides. This cellular immune response, which is mostly directed at the relatively invariant internal virus proteins (Gotch *et al*, 1987), can provide a degree of cross-protection and can protect individuals from severe infection if they have good T-cell memory from an earlier infection (McMichael *et al*, 1983). The specificity of these immune responses is influenced by HLA type, and influenza virus may select out HLA types associated with favourable immune responses. Such selective forces have not been described for influenza, because opportunities for this type of study have not presented themselves. (This might be possible in the early stages of the next pandemic.) However, there is good evidence from Hill's study of malaria, that the HLA type B53 offers considerable protection against fatal (if untreated) severe malaria of young children (Hill *et al*, 1991). Probably, as a consequence, HLA B53 has been selected as a common HLA type in West Africa. It is found in 25% of the population in The Gambia but in less than 1% of the population of Western Europe. It is quite possible that similar selective pressures have been and are being exerted by influenza.

Human immunodeficiency virus (HIV)

HIV is an example of a virus which persists, but which also varies dramatically when different isolates are compared (Korber *et al*, 1995). In addition to the two main types, HIV-1 and HIV-2, there are multiple subtypes, particularly in the case of HIV-1. These subtypes or clades, (A–J), have different though overlapping geographical distributions (Louwagie *et al*, 1993). There is great variability within each clade, and it is normal to find many variants, a quasi-species swarm, within each infected patient. The reasons for this variability are clear given the considerable and continuous turnover of virus (Ho *et al*, 1995; Wei *et al*, 1995). Even in patients with relatively low viral loads, there may be 10^9–10^{10} viruses produced every day. The viral genome is 10^4 nucleotides long and so even with a relatively modest virus mutation rate of 10^{-5}, one in 10 viruses will contain a mutation. In fact, mutation rates are probably higher and the actual figure is closer to one new mutation per viral genome. Therefore, 10^8–10^9 new mutants are made every day, which covers every single possibility (3×10^4) many times, and most or all double mutants (9×10^8). The mutation rate is relatively high because of errors in reverse transcription and lack of editing of RNA copying (Coffin, 1995). The majority of viral mutants are defective, so there is a considerable load of cells infected with defective provirus and of virus particles that are unable to infect and replicate. However, a subset are functional and can compete as viable viruses. They offer a capacity to evade immune responses, as both the antibody and T-cell immune responses focus on small parts of the viral structure. Critical antibody epitopes which result in neutralisation involve relatively few amino acids, e.g. the apical 12 amino acids of the V3 loop (Nara *et al*, 1990; Arendrup *et al*, 1993; Kliks *et al*, 1993; Burns and Desrosiers, 1994; Moore *et al*, 1994).

However, many of the epitopes are conformational, though small. CTL tend to focus on only a handful of epitopes, and sometimes only one; each of which is only only eight to 10 amino acids long (Falk *et al*, 1991). There is good evidence now that both antibody and cytotoxic T-lymphocytes select virus variants during the course of infection. The strongest neutralizing antibody response is directed at the V3 loop, which is the most variable part of the viral envelope. During virus infection, the V3 loop evolves as a result of antibody selection (Nara *et al*, 1990; Arendrup *et al*, 1993; Kliks *et al*, 1993; Burns and Desrosiers, 1994; Moore *et al*, 1994). It has recently been found that the envelope, including the V3 region, controls tropism by selecting different co-receptors on lymphocytes and macrophages, CCR5 or CXCR4 (Choe *et al*, 1996, Doranz *et al*, 1996, Dragic *et al*, 1996), thus adding another dimension to the selective forces at play, but neither is mutually exclusive. The CTL response tends to focus on internal virus proteins as well as the envelope, and there are now well described examples in which strong CTL responses have selected viral variants. Such escapes can occur in the acute phase of infection (Borrow *et al*, 1997; Price *et al*, 1997), when the CTL response is highly active in bringing virus load down to moderate levels, during the middle phase of the infection when virus load is fairly stable (Phillips *et al*, 1991; Nowak *et al*, 1995), and in late infection when there can be a sudden rise in virus load and development of AIDS (Goulder *et al*, 1997). A balance must exist between the capacity of the immune response to select, the tendency of the virus to mutate and the viability of individual escape mutants. As virus escapes immune responses, the immune system can respond by reacting to epitopes in other regions of the virus. However, this capacity is not infinite and the cost may well be an increased virus load because the evolving immune response is directed at increasingly suboptimal epitopes. This means that the virus can be controlled, but with an increasing virus load and more rapid loss of CD4-positive T-cells. When CD4-positive T-cells fail, all immune responses are impaired, including CTL which are dependent for their maintenance on T-helper cell cytokine production (Walter *et al*, 1995). Nowak (Nowak *et al*, 1991; Nowak and McMichael, 1995) has suggested that there is a diversity threshold at which point the immune response fails and the virus escapes completely. Although this hypothesis has attracted a lot of criticism (Wolinsky *et al*, 1996), the concept is logical provided it is realized that the thresholds may differ for different patients, and that the threshold may be reached more rapidly when the CD4 count (and function) has declined to levels at which the immune system can no longer react to new variants.

It is noteworthy that HIV has not diversified in the population to give an ever-expanding continuum of virus variants with no recognisable subtypes. In fact, it has been shown that the viral envelope in the early stage of the infection is relatively homogeneous (Holmes *et al*, 1992). Furthermore, the CCR5 receptor is essential for infection, because homozygotes for a deletion in CCR5 are highly resistant to all forms of HIV infection (Paxton *et al*, 1996). However, a case has been reported recently of an HIV-positive individual homozygous for the CCR5 mutation that abrogates expression (Biti *et al*, 1997). These observations imply a bottle-neck (or bottle-necks) that may force the virus back towards a mean, or one of a small number of means, as in clades A–J. In sequencing HIV variants in individual patients, it is quite striking that each patient has virus very close to the consensus sequence in all of the virus proteins for the infecting clade from which many of the variants present seem to derive.

The variation in HIV, occurring in each patient and selected by immune responses, is very likely to play a major part in the pathogenesis of the infection. Failure to control the virus is the critical, unique, feature of this infection. The epidemiological importance of the variability is considerable. For instance, it is possible that different clades behave in different ways (Soto-Ramirez *et al*, 1996). The heterosexual spread of HIV-1, the higher rates of mother–baby transmission and the shorter lifespan of HIV-infected patients seen in Africa and Asia than elsewhere may in part be explained if viruses of some clades are more aggressive (Soto-Ramirez *et al*, 1996). However, the influence of other well known epidemiological factors need to be disentangled, including nutritional state, and the presence of other infections, especially other sexually transmitted infections.

HIV is a recent infection and it is too early to demonstrate its influence on the genetic make-up of particular human populations, although with time one might expect the gene frequency of the CCR5 deletion to rise. Conversely, the effect of the host genetic variability on the nature of the prevalent viruses may emerge as an important factor. There is a good prior example of this phenomenon in the case of Epstein–Barr virus (EBV). EBV also infects and persists; it evades immune control by downregulating expression of most virus gene products in persistently infected cells (Young *et al*, 1989), and one of those remaining impairs processing of viral proteins (antigens) within these cells (Levitskaya *et al*, 1995). Infected people with the HLA type A11 in Western countries make very potent CTL responses to this virus. Although the virus is an episomal DNA virus, some variability does occur and it is striking that in south-east Asia, where HLA A11 is common (30–50% of some populations), the dominant peptide epitope in EBV that binds to HLA A11 to stimulate CTL responses is altered by one amino acid, so that it no longer binds to HLA A11 (de Campos-Lima *et al*, 1994). It appears, therefore, that this variant of the virus, having mutated to evade this immune response, has spread throughout the whole population. Such a mechanism could account for the different geographical distribution of the different HIV clades but, if so, such selection would have had to be extremely rapid and to have occurred at multiple sites in the virus.

Conclusion

The interrelationship between differing susceptibility of human populations to virus infection and variability in viruses, is extremely complex and at an early stage of investigation. The examples discussed here illustrate the complexity of the problem, but do show that selection of one by the other can be demonstrated by careful study. Understanding such interactions is important for our full understanding of epidemic virus infections and is important in designing strategies for their control.

References

Arendrup M, Sonnerborg A, Svennerholm B *et al.* Neutralizing antibody response during human immunodeficiency virus type 1 infection: type and group specificity and viral escape. *Journal of General Virology*, 1993; **74**: 855–863

Askonas BA, McMichael AJ, Webster RG. The immune response to influenza virus and the problem of protection against infection. In: Beare AS (ed), *Basic and Applied Influenza Research*. Boca Raton: CRC Press, 1982, pp 157–188

Biti R, Ffrench R, Young J, Bennetts B, Stewart G. HIV-1 infection in an individual homozygous for the CCR5 deletion allele. *Nature Medicine*, 1997; **3**: 252–253

Bjorkman PJ, Saper MA, Samraoui B, Bennett WS, Strominger J, Wiley DC. Structure of the human class I histocompatibility antigen, HLA-A2. *Nature*, 1987; **329**: 506–511

Borrow P, Lewicki H, Wei X *et al.* Antiviral pressure exerted by HIV-1 specific cytotoxic T lymphocytes (CTLs) during primary infection demonstrated by rapid selection of CTL escape virus. *Nature Medicine*, 1997; **3**: 205–211

Burns DP, Desrosiers RC. Envelope sequence variation, neutralizing antibodies, and primate lentivirus persistence. *Current Topics in Microbiology and Immunology*, 1994; **188**: 185–219

Choe H, Farzan M, SunY *et al.* The β-chemokine receptors CCR3 and CCR5 facilitate infection by primary HIV-1 isolates. *Cell*, 1996; **85**: 1135–1148

Claas ECJ, Osterhaus AD, van Beek R *et al.* Human influenza A H5N1 virus related to a highly pathogenic avian influenza virus. *Lancet*, 1998, **351**: 472–477.

Coffin JM. HIV population dynamics *in vivo*: implications for genetic variation, pathogenesis, and therapy. *Science*, 1995; **267**: 483–489

de Campos-Lima PO, Levitsky V, Brooks J *et al.* T cell responses and virus evolution: Loss of HLA A11-restricted CTL epitopes in EBV isolates from highly A11-positive populations by selective mutation of anchor residues. *Journal of Experimental Medicine*, 1994; **179**: 1297–1305

Doranz BJ, Rucker J, Yi Y *et al.* A dual-tropic primary HIV-1 isolate that uses Fusin and the β-chemokine receptors CKR-5, CKR-3 and CKR-2b as fusion cofactors. *Cell*, 1996; **85**: 1149–1158

Dragic T, Litwin V, Allaway GP *et al.* HIV-1 entry into CD4+ cells is mediated by the chemokine receptor CC-CKR-5. *Nature*, 1996; **381**: 667–673

Falk K, Rotzschke O, Stevanovic S, Jung G, Rammensee HG. Allele-specific motifs revealed by sequencing of self-peptides eluted from MHC molecules. *Nature*, 1991; **351**: 290–296

Glass RI, Brann EA, Slade JD *et al.* Community-wide surveillance of influenza after outbreaks due to H3N2 (A/Victoria/75 and A/Texas/77) and H1N1 (A/USSR/77) influenza viruses, Mercer County, New Jersey, 1978. *Journal of Infectious Disease*, 1978; **138**: 703–706

Gojobori T, Yamaguchi Y, Ikeo K, Mizokami M. Evolution of pathogenic viruses with special reference to the rates of synonymous and nonsynonymous substitutions. *Japanese Journal of Genetics*, 1994; **69**: 481–488

Gotch FM, McMichael AJ, Smith GL, Moss B. Identification of viral molecules recognised by influenza-specific human cytotoxic T lymphocytes. *Journal of Experimental Medicine*, 1987; **165**: 408–416

Goulder PJ, Phillips RE, Colbert RA *et al.* Late escape from an immunodominant cytotoxic T-lymphocyte response associated with progression to AIDS. *Nature Medicine*, 1997; **3**: 212–217.

Hill AV, Allsopp CE, Kwiatkowski D *et al.* Common West African HLA antigens are associated with protection from severe malaria. *Nature*, 1991; **352**: 595–600

Ho DD, Neumann AU, Perelson AS, Chen W, Leonard JM, Markowitz M. Rapid turnover of plasma virions and CD4 lymphocytes in HIV-1 infection. *Nature*, 1995; **373**: 123–126

Holmes EC, Zhang LQ, Simmonds P, Ludlam CA, Leigh-Brown AJ. Convergent and divergent sequence evolution in the surface envelope glycoprotein of human immunodeficiency virus type I within a single infected patient. *Proceedings of the National Academy of Sciences of the USA*, 1992; **89**: 4835–4839

Kliks SC, Shioda T, Haigwood NL, Levy JA. V3 variability can influence the ability of an antibody to neutralise or enhance infection by diverse strains of human immunodeficiency virus type 1. *Proceedings of the National Academy of Sciences of the USA*, 1993; **90**: 11 518–11 522

Korber B, Koup R, Walker B, Haynes B, Moore J, Myers G. *HIV Molecular Immunology Database.* Los Alamos, NM 87545: Theoretical Biology and Biophysics Group, Los Alamos National Laboratory, 1995

Levitskaya J, Coram M, Levitsky V *et al.* Inhibition of antigen processing by the internal repeat region of the Epstein–Barr virus nuclear antigen-1. *Nature*, 1995; 375: 685–688

Lightman S, Cobbold S, Waldmann H, Askonas BA. Do L3T4+ T cells act as effector cells in protection against influenza virus infection? *Immunology*, 1987; **62**: 139–144

Louwagie J, McCutchan FE, Peeters M *et al.* Phylogenetic analysis of gag genes from 70 international HIV-1 isolates provides evidence for multiple genotypes. *AIDS*, 1993; **7**: 769–780

McMichael AJ, Gotch FM, Rothbard J. HLA B37 determines an influenza A virus nucleoprotein epitope recognized by cytotoxic T lymphocytes. *Journal of Experimental Medicine*, 1986; **164**: 1397–1406

McMichael AJ, Gotch FM, Noble GR, Beare PA. Cytotoxic T-cell immunity to influenza. *New England Journal of Medicine*, 1983; **309**: 13–17

Moore JP, CaoY, Ho DD, Koup RA. Development of the anti-gp120 antibody response during seroconversion to human immunodeficiency virus type 1. *Journal of Virology*, 1994; **68**: 5142–5155

Morris AG, Lin Y-L, Askonas BA. Immune interferon release when a cloned cytotoxic T cell line meets its correct influenza-infected target cell. *Nature*, 1982; **295**: 150–152

Nara PL, Smit L, Dunlop N *et al.* Emergence of viruses resistant to neutralisation by V3-specific antibodies in experimental human immunodeficiency virus type 1 IIIB infection of chimpanzees. *Journal of Virology*, 1990; **64**: 3779–3791

Noble GR. Epidemiological and clinical aspects of influenza. In: Beare AS (ed), *Basic and Applied Influenza Research.* Boca Raton: CRC Press, 1982, pp 11–50

Nowak MA, McMichael AJ. How HIV defeats the immune system. *Scientific American*, 1995; **273**: 58–65

Nowak MA, Anderson RM, McLean AR, Wolfs TF, Goudsmit J, May RM. Antigenic diversity thresholds and the development of AIDS. *Science*, 1991; **254**: 963–969

Nowak MA, May RM, Phillips RE *et al.* Antigenic oscillations and shifting immunodominance in HIV-1 infections. *Nature*, 1995; **375**: 606–611

Paxton WA, Martin SR, Tse D *et al.* Relative resistance to HIV-1 infection of CD4 lymphocytes from persons who remain uninfected despite multiple high-risk sexual exposures. *Nature Medicine*, 1996; **2**: 412–417

Phillips RE, Rowland-Jones SL, Nixon DF. Human immunodeficiency virus genetic variation that can escape cytotoxic T cell recognition. *Nature*, 1991; **354**: 453–459

Price DA, Goulder PJR, Klenerman P *et al.* Positive selection of HIV-1 cytotoxic T lymphocyte escape variants during primary infection. *Proceedings of the National Academy of Sciences of the USA*, 1997; **94**: 1890–1895

Soto-Ramirez LE, Renjifo B, McLane MF *et al.* HIV-1 Langerhans' cell tropism associated with heterosexual transmission of HIV. *Science*, 1996; **271**: 1291–1293

Taubenberger JK, Reid AH, Krafft AE, Bijwaard KE, Fanning TG. Initial genetic characterization of the 1918 'Spanish' influenza virus. *Science*, 1997; **275**: 1793–1796

Townsend AR, Rothbard J, Gotch FM, Bahadur B, Wraith D, McMichael AJ. The epitopes of influenza nucleoprotein recognized by cytotoxic T lymphocytes can be defined with short synthetic peptides. *Cell*, 1986; **44**: 959–968

Walter EA, Greenberg PD, Gilbert MJ *et al.* Reconstitution of cellular immunity against cytomegalovirus in recipients of allogeneic bone marrow by transfer of T-cell clones from the donor. *New England Journal of Medicine*, 1995; **333**: 1038–1044

Webster RG, Laver WG, Air GM, Schild GC. Molecular mechanisms of variation in influenza viruses. *Nature*, 1982; **296**: 115–121

Wei X, Ghosh SK, Taylor ME *et al.* Viral dynamics in human immunodeficiency virus type 1 infection. *Nature*, 1995; **373**: 117–122

Wiley DC, Wilson IA, Skehel JJ. Structural identification of the antibody-binding sites of Hong Kong influenza haemagglutinin and their involvement in antigenic variation. *Nature*, 1981; **289**: 373–378

Wolinsky SM, Korber BT, Neumann AU *et al.* Adaptive evolution of human immunodeficiency virus-type 1 during the natural course of infection. *Science*, 1996; **272**: 537–542

Yap KL, Ada GL. Cytotoxic T cells in the lungs of mice infected with influenza A virus. *Scandinavian Journal of Immunology*, 1978; **7**: 73–80

Young L, Alfieri C, Henessey K *et al.* Expression of Epstein–Barr virus transformation associated genes in tissues of patients with EBV lymphoproliferative disease. *New England Journal of Medicine*, 1989; **321**: 1080–1085

5 Drug resistance: we may not be able to go back again

Bruce R. Levin

Department of Biology, Emory University, Atlanta, USA

The extensive and increasing use of antibiotics and other antimicrobial agents over the past 60 years can be seen as an evolutionary experiment of extraordinary proportions. These chemicals, which either kill or prevent the replication of micro-organisms, impose an intense selective force not only on their target populations of pathogens, but also on the normally innocent commensal and beneficial microbes that are inadvertently exposed to them. In the presence of these compounds, bacteria, viruses, fungi or protozoa that are resistant to their action have a tremendous selective advantage over those that are susceptible. As a consequence of this not-quite-natural selection, evolution has resulted in almost monotonic increases in the number of species of microbes with resistant members, in the frequency of resistant strains within each species and in the number of different chemical agents to which individual microbes are resistant. Bacteria, viruses, fungi and protozoa resistant to previously effective chemotherapeutic agents may well be the most significant single source of emerging and re-emerging pathogens in the developed and overdeveloped world and the most important infectious threat to the future of human health.

In this chapter, I consider the problem of microbial resistance to chemotherapy from the perspective of population and evolutionary biology. While I provide an overview of the nature and scope of the resistance problem, my primary concern is the future of resistance. Will antimicrobial resistance be an ever-increasing problem and, as has been suggested, are we approaching the end of the era of antimicrobial chemotherapy? Are there ways to stem the tide of evolving resistance? What are the alternatives to antimicrobial chemotherapy as we know it? In this chapter, I concentrate on bacterial resistance to antibiotics, but many of

New and Resurgent Infections: Prediction, Detection and Management of Tomorrow's Epidemics.
Edited by B. Greenwood and K. De Cock.

the processes discussed apply equally to the various forms of chemotherapy employed to treat viral, protozoal and fungal infections.

The nature, dimensions and causes of the problem of antibiotic resistance

As a consequence of the development and production of naturally occurring, synthetic and semisynthetic antibacterial chemotherapeutic agents (antibiotics or drugs for convenience), we have been able to treat successfully almost all of the major bacterial infections of the past. Previously lethal diseases like tuberculosis, dysentery, syphilis, pneumonia, meningitis and typhoid fever can be cured by antibiotic treatment. This is also the case for the debilitating, but usually non-lethal, infections that continually plague us, like gonorrhoea, urinary tract and ear infections. Effective prophylaxis and/or treatment by antimicrobial chemotherapeutic agents is essential to the major achievements of transplant and other surgery as well as to cancer chemotherapy. While antibiotics, and medical interventions in general, have contributed only a modest amount to the dramatic decline in infectious disease mortality during the past 150 years (McKeown, 1976), in the industrialized world at least, our sense of well-being in the face of the threat of bacterial diseases can be attributed to our belief in the availability and efficacy of antimicrobial chemotherapy.

The evolution and spread of drug-resistant pathogens have begun to erode this faith. The mechanisms and inheritance of resistance to antibiotics are diverse. Bacteria can acquire resistance to antibiotics by four main mechanisms: (i) modification of the target of the drug, (ii) a change in the permeability of the cell to that drug, (iii) activation of pumps that expel drugs that enter the cell, and (iv) the production of enzymes or other compounds that denature or otherwise inactivate or detoxify drugs (Greenwood, 1995). These resistance mechanisms can be acquired by simple mutations of chromosomal genes in otherwise susceptible cells or by gene transfer from other, resistant, bacteria. The latter can be achieved by transformation, the acquisition of free DNA carrying these genes; by conjugation, the receipt of a resistance-encoding accessory genetic element, a plasmid or transposon; or by transduction, infection by a bacteriophage carrying the resistance gene. Plasmid-mediated resistance is the most ominous of these mechanisms. These autonomously replicating and infectiously transmitted DNA molecules may carry genes (transposons) for resistance to five or more antibiotics. Many plasmids and some transposons code for the conjugative pili and other machinery necessary for infectious transfer of DNA to bacteria of the same and, occasionally, different species. Plasmids and transposons that lack the capacity for self-transmission can be picked up, mobilised, and transmitted by conjugative machinery of self-transmissible plasmids (Falkow, 1975; Davies and Smith, 1978).

The human costs and dimensions of the resistance problem

Resistance can prevent or postpone a successful outcome to chemotherapy and thereby increase the morbidity or rates of mortality associated with infections. In the presence of resistance, antibiotic treatment can also be the direct cause of disease. Thus, resistant pathogens may be able to colonize a host and/or increase in density in a host as a result of previous administration of antibiotics which cause the demise of the susceptible populations of commensal microbes that normally prevent colonization or multiplication of the pathogen. Despite the clear potential for resistance to increase the severity of otherwise treatable bacterial infections, illustrated in several case studies (CDC, 1993a), the absolute magnitude of the excess morbidity or mortality attributable to resistance has yet to be calculated. Part of the problem in obtaining these estimates lies in the difficulty of doing case-controlled studies of treated patients infected with susceptible or resistant bacteria (Holmberg *et al*, 1987; Edmond *et al*, 1996). Another problem is that most antibiotic therapy is empiric, treatment being given in the absence of direct information about the microbe responsible for symptoms or its susceptibility to drugs. One mathematical model has tried to predict the economic cost of antibiotic resistance (Phelps, 1989), but the assumptions of that model are very restrictive (hard to justify), and the range of the predicted costs of resistance is more than two orders of magnitude, 0.1 billion to 30 billion a year, in 1979 US dollars. While there may be doubt about the exact costs attributable to resistance, it is clear that the human costs of resistance can be substantial and are rising as resistance becomes more widespread. The rate at which new antibiotics are put on the market is declining, while bacteria are acquiring resistance to existing compounds at increasing rates (Cohen, 1992; 1994; Neu, 1994; Fraimow and Abrutyn, 1995). The frequencies of resistant isolates and the number of different antibiotics to which species and individual bacteria are resistant have been increasing almost monotonically in some of the major community-acquired and hospital-acquired (nosocomial) pathogens (see Figure 5.1a, b). There are already strains of at least two groups of bacteria, *Mycobacterium tuberculosis* and *Enterococcus* (a major nosocomial pathogen), that are resistant to virtually all formerly effective antibiotics (Bloom and Murray, 1992; CDC, 1993b). It is reasonable to anticipate that in the not-too-distant future, more species of bacteria will evolve strains refractory to all available antibiotics.

The evolution of resistance is a direct consequence of antibiotic use. Evolutionary biologists are often (and sometimes justifiably) accused of story-telling when they speculate about the selection forces responsible for a particular adaptive character (Gould and Lewontin, 1979). In the case of drug resistance, however, evidence that the selection force is frequency of exposure resulting from the human use and overuse of antimicrobial chemotherapy and prophylaxis is overwhelming. Chromosomal resistance is acquired by modification of genes responsible for other functions and, as such, is commonly associated with some

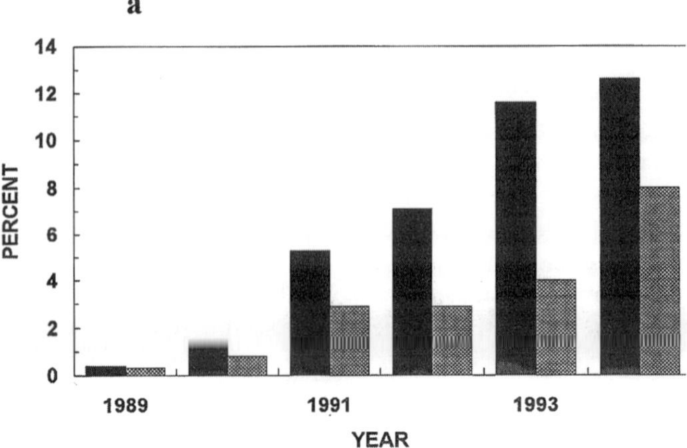

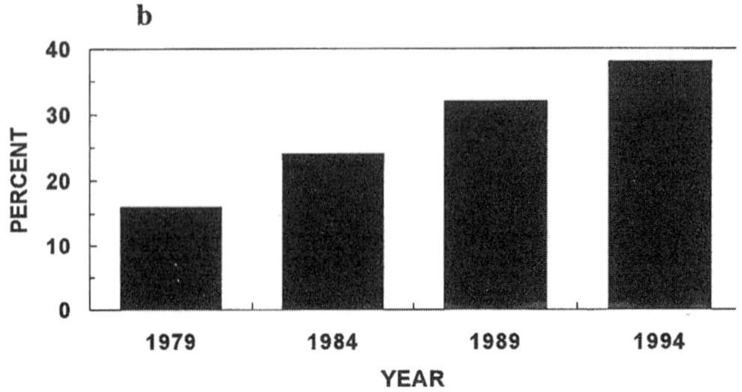

Figure 5.1 (a) Percentage of nosocomial enterococci reported as resistant to vancomycin isolated from infections in patients in intensive-care units, ICUs, (black bars) and non-ICUs (grey bars), by year. National Nosocomial Infection Surveillance System, 1989 to 31 March 1993 (CDC, 1993a). (b) Percentage of Salmonella isolates resistant to one or more antimicrobial agents in four prospective national surveys conducted at 5-year intervals. Adapted, in part from Cohen (1992) and extended with additional data provided by M. L. Cohen (Division of Bacterial and Mycotic Diseases, US Centers for Disease Control and Prevention)

cost to the fitness of the bacteria in the absence of the antibiotic (Schrag and Perrot, 1996). Resistance plasmids often engender a cost on the host bacterium as well (Levin, 1980; Levin and Stewart, 1980; Bouma and Lenski, 1988; Simonsen, 1992). In the absence of drug-mediated selection, bacteria carrying these otherwise deleterious genes and plasmids would never thrive.

The plasmids and transposons responsible for accessory element-encoded resistance almost certainly existed before the antibiotic era (Datta and Hughes, 1983; Hughes and Datta, 1983). This is likely also to be the case for at least some of the plasmid-borne resistance genes (Davies *et al*, 1977; Davies and Gray, 1984). However, the present distribution and frequency of these resistance plasmids and transposons are a direct product of antibiotic-mediated selection for bacteria carrying these elements. These plasmids acquired resistance to individual drugs in much the same order in which these drugs were released onto the market. Moreover, these resistance plasmids increased in frequency and spread with increasing use of these drugs (Falkow, 1975; Levy, 1992). The molecular evolution of the enzymes, β-lactamases, responsible for resistance to the penicillins and cephalosporins can be followed. As new and modified β-lactam antibiotics were introduced, the genes coding for these enzymes changed to generate resistance to these newer antibiotics (Reguera *et al*, 1991; Blazquez *et al*, 1993; Blazquez *et al*, 1995). A final argument that supports the contention that the resistance problem is a direct product of antibiotic-mediated selection is that, in the main, the frequency of drug-resistant microbes is directly proportional to the extent to which those drugs are used in a given area. Countries or regions of countries that employ greater than average amounts of antibiotics have higher frequencies of resistance (Nissinen *et al*, 1995, Arason *et al*, 1996) and the frequency of resistance increases with the amount of time that these agents are used (Nissinen *et al*, 1995).

The population genetics of antibiotic resistance

Is antibiotic resistance likely to be reversible by reducing the rate at which the relevant drugs are employed? On first consideration, the arguments in support of this optimistic interpretation are compelling. In the absence of the selecting drugs, resistance is likely to engender a fitness cost or, at least, it is unlikely to confer an advantage on a microbe. Moreover, for most species of microbes, resistance is a new character and the fitness burdens it imposes on a microbe are unlikely to have been eliminated by subsequent evolution. As a result, if the rate of antibiotic use is reduced, sensitive microbes should have a net advantage and the frequency of resistance should wane. While this intuitive interpretation is, in principle, correct, a more formal (mathematical) consideration of the population genetics of resistance and experimental studies of the cost and modification of the cost of resistance comes to a more pessimistic conclusion. Resistance can be sustained by a balance between selection forces. Even in the most intense situations of antibiotic use, only a fraction of the population of microbes are subject to antibiotic-mediated selection. Under some conditions, this can result in a stable equilibrium in which the population of microbes at large is polymorphic and includes substantial frequencies of susceptible as well as resistant bacteria. Equilibria of this type are anticipated in the case of commensal, but occasionally pathogenic, microbes such as *E. coli*, *Haemophilus influenzae*, *Neisseria meningiditis*, the streptococci and staphylococci.

We have used a mathematical model (Levin *et al*, 1997) to study the consequences of antibiotic-mediated selection on these sustained, commensal, populations. Our model assumes an array of hosts that all maintain populations of these commensal microbes and exchange them through a common reservoir at rates g and f per day, respectively. In the absence of antibiotic-mediated selection, resistant microbes have a selective disadvantage, s $(0<s<1)$, such that their growth rate, fitness, relative to susceptible microbes is $(1-s):1$. Hosts are treated with antibiotics at a rate T per year. We assume that once a host is treated all drug sensitive microbes in that host are eliminated. That this is likely to be the case is supported by the personal observation that after a single day of oral tetracycline treatment, the frequency of resistance in my *E. coli* flora rose from approximately 2×10^{-3} to 1.0 (all of the *E. coli* I recovered were resistant to tetracycline).

Simulation studies using this model indicate that even when the rate of antibiotic use is low and the fitness costs of resistance moderate, the frequency of resistance can be substantial. The model indicates that a 2% reduction in the fitness of resistant microbes relative to susceptible, and with each host undergoing antibiotic treatment on average every second year, the anticipated equilibrium frequency of resistance is about 30%. With treatment twice a year, the anticipated equilibrium frequency of resistance exceeds 60%. Rates of antibiotic treatment of this magnitude are not unprecedented, especially for children. In their study of penicillin-resistant pneumococci in children in Iceland, Arason and colleagues (Arason *et al*, 1996) found that children under six years old were, on average taking between 1.1 to 2.6 courses of antibiotics a year while those under two years of age received treatment twice as frequently.

A quick ascent and slow decline

While the above equilibrium theory indicates that a reduction in the rate of antibiotic treatment will be followed by a decline in the frequency of resistance, it does not provide information about the rate of that decline. There is good reason to assume that the rate at which resistance will wane in the absence of antibiotics will be substantially lower than that at which it ascends when antibiotics are being employed. In accord with population genetic theory, the rate of increase in the frequency of a gene is anticipated to be directly proportional to the intensity of selection favouring that gene (Crow and Kimura, 1971). It is reasonable to anticipate that when antibiotics are employed, the intensity of selection for resistance will be high, while in the absence of antibiotics, the intensity of selection favouring drug susceptibility (against resistance) will be relatively low. The consequences of this are illustrated in Figure 5.2, where the rate of change in the frequency of a gene with different intensities of selection is presented. In this

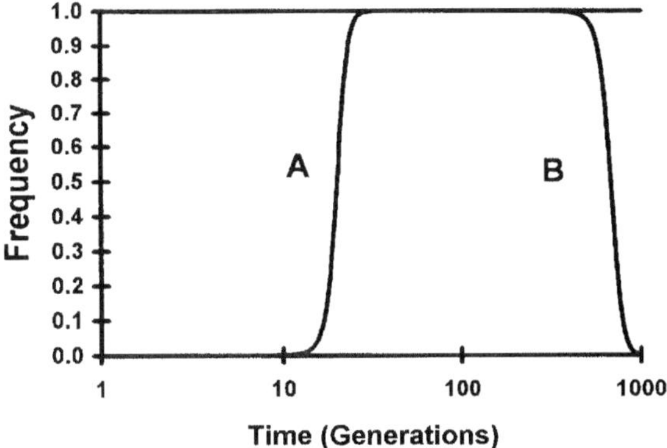

Figure 5.2 Changes in the frequency of a drug-resistant strain calculated from the formula for selection in a haploid population with discrete generations, $Dp = pqs/(1 - qs)$ where p is the frequency of the favoured gene (clone), $q = (1 - p)$ the frequency of the allele (clone) which is being selected against and s the selection coefficient, $0 < s < 1$. In the situation represented by line A, the resistant clone has a 50% fitness advantage, $s = 0.50$, relative to the susceptible. In the situation represented by line B, the resistant clone has a 2% fitness disadvantage, $s = 0.02$, relative to the susceptible. In both cases, the initial frequency of the favoured gene (clone) is 10^{-6}

example, it is assumed that resistance confers a 50% selective advantage in the presence of an antibiotic and a 2% disadvantage in the absence of that antibiotic. In both cases, the initial frequency of the favoured gene is 10^{-6}.

Figure 5.2 also illustrates another prediction from classical population genetics theory—the slow start phenomenon. The change in the frequency of resistance is sigmoid. The maximum rate of change in frequency is seen when the sensitive and resistant genes are equally frequent. When a resistant strain is rare, the rate of increase in its frequency is low. Even when resistance has been in a population for some time and is continuously increasing in frequency, it takes some time before it reaches frequencies where it is likely to be recognized in clinical samples, on the order of 1%. However, once resistance is at detectable frequencies, and exposure to antibiotics continues, the rate of increase in its frequency is rapid. This has a very practical implication for hospitals or other closed settings where resistance to a specific antibiotic is believed to have been controlled by terminating the use of that compound. Under these conditions it is critical to sample extensively and selectively to be sure that the frequency of resistance to that drug is close to zero before resuming its use.

For situations where resistance is acquired by the receipt of a plasmid or other accessory element, the time before it is observed in a particular species or lineage of bacteria is likely to be even longer than that anticipated by the simple population genetics model considered in Figure 5.2, in which the resistant genotype is already present. In the former case, the plasmid or other accessory element has to acquire the resistance genes (Levin, 1995), make its way from its ancestral species or lineage to that under consideration, and be expressed in that bacterium. This can take time. For example, most of the 30 years between the introduction of vancomycin and the first clinical observation of vancomycin resistance is likely to have been taken up by the evolution of the plasmid responsible for this resistance from a yet-to-be determined source, and its movement to the species in which it was detected. If this is correct, the rate at which new species and lineages of bacteria acquire resistance to this antibiotic is likely to increase now that Van resistance plasmids have been observed in pathogens, and are becoming increasingly common. Rumours of the first confirmed sightings of vancomycin-resistant *Staphylococcus aureus* are circulating.

The situation considered in Figure 5.2 assumes purely directional selection in which either resistant or susceptible microbes have a net advantage. As noted above, there are conditions, at least in the case of commensal microbes, in which stable polymorphisms with resistant and susceptible strains are anticipated, with the frequency of resistance being proportional to the rate of antibiotic use (Levin *et al*, 1997). Recently, Stewart *et al* (1997), using a variant of the model employed by Levin and collaborators, considered the rate of change in the frequency of resistance with incremental changes in the rates of treatment. According to this model, a 10-fold drop in the rate of treatment, from 2 per year to 0.2 per year, would reduce the equilibrium frequency of resistance from about 0.37 to 0.06, assuming that resistance engenders a 1% cost in fitness. This change would be anticipated to occur in about 22 weeks, assuming a 40-hour generation time for the bacteria.

The epidemiology of acute infections

The epidemiology of resistance for acute infections that are cleared following treatment is likely to be different from that described above for sustained populations of commensal microbes. Some models of treatment of acute infections suggest that stable polymorphisms with susceptible and resistant bacteria are possible (Massad *et al*, 1993). The conditions needed for this to obtain have to be superimposed on the model and, in that sense, are restrictive. Under more general conditions, the compartment models used for developing this theory suggest that there would be threshold concentrations of antibiotics, above which selection would favour resistance and below which susceptible strains would have an advantage (Antia *et al*, in preparation). In this situation, the population will be approaching outcomes where there are only resistant or sensitive microbes. In these acute infection models, the fitness costs associated with resistance are expressed as either lower rates of transmission, or higher rates of clearance in the absence of treatment.

Experimental studies of the cost of resistance

Fundamental to the premise that the frequency of resistance will decline with reductions in the rate of use of antimicrobials, is the assumption that resistance engenders a cost in the fitness of microbes. The costs of resistance in the absence of drugs might be manifest in a variety of ways: reduced rates of growth, increased rates of mortality, reduced competitive performance in a host or the external environment, lower rates of infectious transmission, lower rates of colonization, or higher rates of clearance in untreated infected hosts. Of these different components of fitness, population growth, competitive performance and mortality rates are most readily estimated experimentally. As noted earlier, there is evidence for these kinds of fitness costs for chromosomal and plasmid-encoded resistance in bacteria (Levin, 1980; Bouma and Lenski, 1988; Simonsen, 1992; Schrag and Perrot, 1996) and for resistance to protease inhibitors in HIV (Borman *et al*, 1996). There is also evidence that exposure to antiviral drugs reduces the virulence of herpes viruses (Coen, 1991). Although it would seem probable that reduced virulence is reflected as a fitness cost, the relationship between virulence and the fitness of microbes is not clear (Levin, 1996).

Despite these examples of fitness costs associated with resistance, it is presently not known how frequently resistance impairs the fitness of a microbe or the magnitude of those costs. For example, we have been unable to detect fitness costs for chromosomal mutations to naladixic acid resistance in *E. coli* maintained in glucose-limited minimal medium.

Even when drug resistance engenders a fitness cost, the magnitude of that cost is likely to wane as a consequence of subsequent evolution (Levin and Lenski, 1983). The logic behind this prediction is straightforward. In the presence of the drug, resistance would be favoured but so would mutations that reduced the fitness cost associated with this resistance. This can happen more rapidly than might be anticipated. Thus, in a study of the adaptation by *E. coli* to the fitness associated with the carriage of a plasmid bearing tetracycline and chloramphenicol resistance, Bouma and Lenski (1988) observed reductions in those costs within 500 generations in serial transfer culture. Furthermore, the strain that evolved in these experiments was more fit when it carried the plasmid than when it did not.This compensatory evolution was obtained by mutation(s) in the host chromosomes, rather than the plasmid, and involved a response to the tetracycline resistance region carried on the plasmid (Lenski *et al*, 1994).

A further example of adaptation to reduce the cost of a resistance-encoding plasmid was observed by Modi and Adams (1991). In their case, this adaptation to the cost of plasmid carriage occurred in chemostat culture in the absence of antibiotic-mediated selection and involved changes in both the chromosome and plasmid, i.e. coevolution. However, in this situation, part of the adaptation involved the loss of its ampicillin resistance transposon by the plasmid (J. Adams, personal communication). More recently, Schrag and Perrot (1996) observed adaptation to the substantial fitness cost associated with the ribosomal mutations responsible for resistance to streptomycin, rpsL, in *E. coli.* This fitness cost was associated with a reduction in the rate of protein elongation during translation. In their evolution experiments, clones carrying second-site compensatory mutations dominated cultures within 180 generations. These compensatory mutations evolved in the absence of streptomycin and returned the rate of protein elongation to apparently normal levels, without reducing the level of resistance to streptomycin. The fitness of the evolved rpsL strains was less than that of their streptomycin-sensitive ancestors, but substantially greater than that of the resistant mutants from which they evolved. Borman and colleagues (1996) also observed compensatory evolution rather than reversion to sensitivity in their *in vitro* study of HIV resistant to a protease inhibitor. Although their tissue culture medium did not contain the antiviral drug, both the fitness of the resistant HIV and the level of resistance increased in the course of passage in that medium.

Compensatory evolution that reduces the cost of drug resistance necessarily engenders changes in the genetic background of the microbe beyond those associated with resistance itself. It is possible that, as a consequence of these changes, microbes with this evolved genetic background, sensitive revertants, or plasmid-free segregants, may have a disadvantage relative to their resistant progenitors. This is what we observed for the streptomycin-resistant rpsL *E. coli* generated in the study by Schrag and Perrot (1996) described above. When unevolved streptomycin-resistant cells are made susceptible, by transducing an rpsL$^+$ allele, they are more fit than the corresponding resistant transductants. The opposite occurs when the same genetic manipulation is done with the rpsL strains with the fitness-compensating, second-site mutation. These evolved streptomycin-sensitive strains have a marked disadvantage relative to the resistant (Schrag *et al*, unpublished work). One interpretation of this result is that this evolved, resistant lineage would be unable to return to drug sensitivity. That is, at least two separate genetic changes would be required for the bacterium to return to wild-type, with each single change imposing a disadvantage in the absence of the selecting drug. This interpretation can also be applied to the studies of adaptation to plasmid carriage studies undertaken by Lenski and colleagues (Bouma and Lenski, 1988; Lenski *et al*, 1994) as well as the HIV protease inhibitor studies done by Borman *et al* (1996). Evolved, fitness-compensated cells that lose the resistance plasmid, or resistant HIV that reverts to more susceptible states, would have a disadvantage relative to resistant. A general extrapolation from these experiments is that although resistance may initially impair the fitness of microbes, in this environment where antimicrobial agents are common, these microbes are likely to adapt to these fitness costs, possibly to the point where they are negligible.

The future of the resistance problem

From a public health perspective it is difficult to interpret the results of these studies of the population genetics of resistance in an optimistic light. They suggest that, even if we reduce the rate at which we use existing antimicrobial agents, the frequency of resistance to those compounds will not decline very rapidly, if at all, and that unless usage stops completely, the sustained frequency of resistance will remain substantial. This interpretation is based primarily on theoretical considerations and laboratory experiments, and it is possible that in reality the frequency of drug-resistant microbes will decline under broader conditions and at greater rates than those predicted by this simple theory and laboratory experiments.

When declines in the frequency of resistance are observed following a reduction in antibiotic use, it is critical that their nature is carefully documented. They could, for example, be reflections of changes in the clonal distribution of the bacterial population that have little, if anything at all, to do with antibiotic resistance or patterns of antibiotic use. Of particular importance in evaluating declines in frequencies of antibiotic resistance in association with reduced antimicrobial use is to ascertain, with the aid of molecular or other data, whether all resistant species and lineages of microbes exposed to that antibiotic also decline in frequency.

One of the most compelling lines of evidence that resistance will not wane rapidly is the existence, in contemporary populations of bacteria, of lineages resistant to drugs that were commonly used in the past but which are currently used only rarely to treat human infections. For example, in a study of the frequency of resistance in the aerobic, enteric flora of infants in a day-care centre, BassamTomeh (unpublished results) found that approximately 25% of these bacteria were resistant to streptomycin (>20 μg/ml) and that two out of the 25 children studied carried bacteria resistant to chloramphenicol. These antibiotics have not been in common use for more than 25 years and do not show cross-resistance to antimicrobials in current use. Resistance to these drugs may be maintained by associated linkage selection of plasmids coding for resistance to antibiotics in current use or by selection resulting from the non-clinical use of these compounds. Streptomycin, for example, is used to prevent bacteria-mediated blemishing of pears and other fruit.

Even if reducing antibiotic use does lead to substantial declines in the frequency of resistant microbes, persuading people to use these agents less frequently will not be an easy task. There are three powerful forces working against this kind of social change. The first, and perhaps most important, factor are the patients being treated. Antibiotic resistance is, in the main, a community, rather than an individual, problem. The tragedy of the commons (Hardin, 1968) prevails; individuals gain while the collective loses. As long as the frequency of resistance remains relatively low, it will affect the course of treatment of few individuals. This is particular true for the treatment of community-acquired, rather than in-hospital-acquired infections. In the community, most treatment is empiric and given in the absence of direct evidence that a bacterial infection, much less one susceptible to antibiotics, is responsible for the symptoms being treated. For the unknown fraction of cases for whom antibiotic treatment is appropriate, the primary aim of this treatment is to reduce morbidity, rather than mortality, as the vast majority of infections are non-lethal and normally cleared without negative, long-term effects. From the perspective of the community, the primary gain of treatment may be some reduction in the transmission of the pathogen and thus the number of new infections (Bonhoeffer *et al*, 1997).

The primary loss to the community of treating individual patients with broad spectrum antibiotics is an increase in the frequency and spread of resistance genes and accessory elements and promotion of the evolution of new plasmids and other accessory elements with resistance genes. The relative magnitudes of these gains and losses are unclear. From the perspective of the patient or his family, losses to the community are abstractions while the true or even perceived gains to the individual are very real.

The second and third human forces that make reductions in antibiotic use problematic relate to physicians and the pharmaceutical industry. The tragedy of the commons applies for them as well. The human need to feel effective may be an even more powerful incentive to use antibiotics than economic considerations. Antibiotics can certainly be effective when they are properly targeted and administered. Under almost all circumstances, prescribing these compounds gives the patient the impression that he or she is being managed effectively and offers a way, satisfying to both parties, to terminate a physician–patient encounter.

The prospect that the problem of drug resistance will become graver if we do not do something about it is the only prudent position. However, I believe that there are a number of ways in which we can prepare for an increase in the frequency and distribution of resistant microbes, in addition to cutting back on the rate of antibiotic use.

Direct identification of the aetiological agent responsible for symptoms and determination of its resistance pattern in an individual patient, is often considered too time-consuming, and results may not become available in time to influence treatment. However, using molecular procedures, it is now becoming possible not only rapidly to identify the microbe responsible for symptoms in an individual patient, but also to determine the resistance pattern of that aetiological agent (see, for example, Kapur *et al*, 1995). While these procedures may be too cumbersome and costly for routine use at present, this may change if the resistance problem does become more acute.

As the resistance problem becomes more serious in the developed world, there will be a increasing incentive for the pharmaceutical industry to develop new antimicrobial agents. Because of the parallel development of rapid diagnostic tools for identifying pathogens, these new drugs could have a narrower spectrum than the antimicrobials currently used for empiric therapy. Genome projects will almost certainly identify additional targets for antimicrobials and thus facilitate the quest for new drugs.

Problems with chemotherapy make prevention, including that achieved with vaccines, an increasingly attractive option. The success of the *Haemophilus influenzae* conjugate vaccine (Barbour, 1996) encourages this approach whilst evaluating the longer-term effects of the wide-scale application of these vaccines (Lipsitch, 1997).

Finally, there are alternative treatment and prophylaxis procedures developed in the past that have been eclipsed by the advent of antibiotics. Included among these are the use of specific antisera, serum therapy or passive immunization (Casadevall and Scharff, 1995) and phage therapy (Lederberg, 1996; Levin and Bull, 1996; Merril *et al*, 1996). While there are many problems with these older alternatives to antibiotics, there is evidence for their efficacy. Moreover, the heyday for serum therapy was long before T-cells and B-cells were recognised or before we had the technology for producing specific antibodies *in vitro*. Similarly, phage therapy was already waning before the Phage School of molecular biology (Cairns *et al*, 1965) was even open. One of the greatest practical problem with these older therapies was their specificity, since one has to know not only the species of microbe responsible for the infection, but the serotype and the spectrum of phage sensitivity, if the microbe was a bacterium. Perhaps that problem could be overcome by rapid molecular diagnostic techniques.

Acknowledgements

I wish to thank Mitchell L. Cohen and his colleagues at the US Centers for Disease Control and Prevention for making their data available to me, and Marc Lipsitch for his insightful and helpful comments on this manuscript. This endeavour, and some of the real work behind it, was supported by a grant from the US National Institutes of Health, GM 33782.

References

Antia R and the EcLF. Epidemiology of drug resistance in acute infections. 1997, in preparation

Arason VA, Kristinsson KG, Sigurdsson JA, Stefansdottir JAG, Molstad S, Gudmundsson S. Do antimicrobials increase the carriage rate of penicillin resistant pneumococci in children? Cross sectional prevalence study. *British Medical Journal*, 1996; **313**: 387–391

Barbour ML. Conjugate vaccines and the carriage of *Haemophilus influenzae* type b. *Emerging Infectious Diseases*, 1996; **2**: 176–182

Blazquez J, Baquero MR, Canton R, Alos I, Baquero F. Characterization of a new TEM-type beta-lactamase resistant to clavulanate, sulbactam, and tazobactam in a clinical isolate of *Escherichia coli. Antimicrobial Agents & Chemotherapy*, 1993; **37**: 2059–2063

Blazquez J, Morosini MI, Negri MC, Gonzalez-Leiza M, Baquero F. Single amino acid replacements at positions altered in naturally occurring extended spectrum TEM beta-lactamases. *Antimicrobial Agents & Chemotherapy*, 1995; **39**: 145–149

Bloom BR, Murray CJ. Tuberculosis—commentary on a reemergent killer. *Science*, 1992; **257**: 1055–1064

Bonhoeffer S, Lipsitch M, Levin BR. Evaluating treatment protocols to prevent antibiotic resistance. *Proceedings of the National Academy of Sciences of the USA*, 1997; in press

Borman AM, Paulous S, Clavel F. Resistance of human immunodeficiency virus type 1 to protease inhibitors: selection of resistance mutations in the presence and absence of the drug. *Journal of General Virology*, 1996; **77**: 419–426

Bouma JE, Lenski RE. Evolution of a bacteria/plasmid association. *Nature*, 1988; **335**: 351–352

Cairns J, Stent G, Watson JD. *Phage and the Origins of Molecular Biology*. Cold Spring Harbor, NY: Cold Spring Harbor Press, 1965

Casadevall A, Scharff MD. Return to the past: the case for antibody based therapies in infectious diseases. *Clinical Infectious Diseases*, 1995; **21**: 150–161

CDC. *National Nosocomial Infections Surveillance System: Methods and Trends in Antimicrobial Resistance*. Atlanta, GA: US Public Health Service, 1993a

CDC. Nosocomial enterococci resistant to vancomycin—United States, 1989–1993. *Morbidity and Mortality Weekly Report*, 1993b; **42**: 597–599

Coen DM. The implications of resistance to antiviral agents for herpesvirus drug targets and drug therapy. *Antiviral Research*, 1991; **15**: 287–300

Cohen ML. Epidemiology of drug-resistance—implications for a post antimicrobial era. *Science*, 1992; **257**: 1050–1055

Cohen ML. Emerging problems of antimicrobial resistance. *Annals of Emergency Medicine*, 1994; **24**: 454–456

Crow JF, Kimura M. *An Introduction to Population Genetics Theory*. New York: Harper Row, 1971

Datta N, Hughes VM. Plasmids of the same Inc groups in enterobacteria before and after the medical use of antibiotics. *Nature*, 1983; **306**: 616–617

Davies J, Courvalin P, Berg D. Thoughts on the origins of resistance plasmids. *Journal of Antimicrobial Chemotherapy*, 1977; **3**: 7–17

Davies J, Gray G. Evolutionary relationships among genes for antibiotic resistance. *Ciba Foundation Symposium*, 1984; **102**: 219–232

Davies J, Smith DI. Plasmid-determined resistance to antimicrobial agents. *Annual Review of Microbiology*, 1978; **32**: 469–518

Edmond MB, Ober JF, Dawson JD, Weinbaum DL, Wenzel RP. Vancomycin resistant enterococcal bacteremia: natural history and attributable mortality. *Clinical Infectious Diseases*, 1996; **23**: 1234–1239

Falkow S. *Infectious Multiple Drug Resistance*. London: Pion Press, 1975

Fraimow HS, Abrutyn E. Pathogens resistant to antimicrobial agents. Epidemiology, molecular mechanisms, and clinical management. *Infectious Disease Clinics of North America*, 1995; **9**: 497–530

Gould SJ, Lewontin RC. The spandrels of San Marco and the Panglossian paradigm: a critique of the adaptationist programme. *Proceedings of the Royal Society, London, Series B*, 1979; **205**: 581–598

Greenwood D (ed). *Antimicrobial Chemotherapy*. Oxford: Oxford University Press, 1995

Hardin G. The tragedy of the commons. The population problem has no technical solution; it requires a fundamental extension in morality. *Science*, 1968; **162**: 1243–1248

Holmberg SD, Solomon SL, Blake PA. Health and economic impacts of antimicrobial resistance. *Reviews of Infectious Disease*, 1987; **9**: 1065–1078

Hughes VM, Datta N. Conjugative plasmids in bacteria of the 'pre-antibiotic' era. *Nature*, 1983; **302**: 725–726

Kapur V, Li LL, Hamrick MR *et al.* Rapid Mycobacterium species assignment and unambiguous identification of mutations associated with antimicrobial resistance in *Mycobacterium tuberculosis* by automated DNA sequencing. *Archives of Pathology and Laboratory Medicine*, 1995; 119: 131–138

Lederberg J. Smaller fleas ... ad infinitum: therapeutic phage redux. *Proceedings of the National Academy of Sciences of the USA*, 1996; **93**: 3167–3168

Lenski RE, Simpson SC, Nguyen TT. Genetic analysis of a plasmid-encoded, host genotype-specific enhancement of bacterial fitness. *Journal of Bacteriology*, 1994; **176**: 3140–3147

Levin BR. Conditions for the existence of R-plasmids in bacterial populations. In: Mitsuhashi S, Rosival L, Krcmery V (eds), *Fourth International Symposium on Antibiotic Resistance.* Berlin: Springer Verlag, 1980, pp 197–202

Levin BR. Conditions for the evolution of multiple antibiotic resistance plasmids: A theoretical and experimental excursion. In: Baumberg S, Young JPW, Saunders SR, Wellington EMH (eds), *The Population Genetics of Bacteria.* Cambridge: Cambridge University Press, 1995, pp 175–192

Levin BR.The evolution and maintenance of virulence in microparasites. *Emerging Infectious Diseases*, 1996; **2**: 93–102

Levin BR, Bull JJ. Phage therapy revisited: the population biology of a bacterial infection and its treatment with bacteriophage and antibiotics. *American Naturalist*, 1996; **147**: 881–898

Levin BR, Lenski RE. Coevolution of bacteria and their viruses and plasmids. In: Futuyama DJ, Slatkin M (eds), *Coevolution.* Sunderland, MA: Sinauer Associates, 1983, pp 99–127

Levin BR, Stewart FM. The population biology of bacterial plasmids: a priori conditions for the existence of mobilizable nonconjugative factors. *Genetics*, 1980; **94**: 425–443

Levin BR, Lipsitch M, Perrot V *et al.* The population genetics of antibiotic resistance. *Clinical Infectious Diseases*, 1997; **24**: S9–16

Levy SB.The Antibiotic Paradox: How Miracle Drugs are Destroying the Miracle. New York: Plenum Press, 1992

Lipsitch M. Vaccination against colonizing bacteria with multiple serotypes. *Proceedings of the National Academy of Sciences of the USA*, 1997; **94**: 6572–6576

Massad E, Lundberg S,Yang HM. Modeling and simulating the evolution of resistance against antibiotics. *International Journal of Biomedical Computing*, 1993; **33**: 65–81

McKeown T. The Role of Medicine: Dream, Mirage or Nemesis. London: Nuffield Provincial Hospitals Trust, 1976

Merril CR, Biswas B, Carlton R *et al.* Long-circulating bacteriophage as antibacterial agents. *Proceedings of the National Academy of Sciences of the USA*, 1996; **93**: 3188–3192

Modi RI, Adams J. Coevolution in bacteria–plasmid populations. *Evolution*, 1991; **45**: 656–667

Neu HC. Emerging trends in antimicrobial resistance in surgical infections. A review. *European Journal of Surgery – Supplement*, 1994; **573**: 7–18

Nissinen A, Gronroos P, Huovinen P *et al.* Development of beta-lactamase-mediated resistance to penicillin in middle-ear isolates of *Moraxella catarrhalis* in Finnish children, 1978–1993. *Clinical Infectious Diseases*, 1995; **21**: 1193–1196

Phelps CE. Bug/drug resistance: sometimes less is more. *Medical Care*, 1989; **27**: 194–203

Reguera JA, Baquero F, Perez-Dias JC, Martinez JL. Factors determining resistance to beta-lactam combined with beta-lactamase inhibitors in *Escherichia coli. Journal of Antimicrobial Chemotherapy*, 1991; **27**: 569–575

Schrag S, Perrot V. Reducing antibiotic resistance. *Nature*, 1996; **28**: 120–121

Simonsen L. The existence conditions for bacterial plasmids. PhD dissertation, University of Massachusetts, Amherst, 1992

Stewart FM, Antia R, Levin BR, Lipsitch M, Mittler JE. The population dynamics of antibiotic resistance II: Analytical theory for sustained populations of bacteria in a population of hosts. *Theoretical Population Biology*, 1997; in press

6 Environmental factors, the immune system and the susceptibility to infection

Luc Kestens and Guido Vanham

Institute of Tropical Medicine, Antwerp, Belgium

Individual susceptibility to infection, disease and death is influenced by various factors such as host genotype, age, psychological state, virulence of the infectious agent and also by ecological, socio-economical and cultural changes. The interplay between these internal and external factors is complex and their relationship to new or resurgent infections is often very poorly understood. It is known that environmental factors can impair the immune system. To what extent these immunological changes modify susceptibility to infection is more difficult to assess and is often speculative.

In this paper, the diversity of the immune response to infectious agents and the impact of external factors such as malnutrition and environmental 'modulators' on these responses are reviewed. As an illustrative example, susceptibility to infection with the human immune deficiency virus (HIV) will be discussed, as well as the way in which this virus, as a recently introduced 'environmental' factor itself, has affected the reappearance of other infectious diseases. HIV changes host susceptibility to tuberculosis, toxoplasmosis and herpes simplex but not to streptococcal infections or malaria. To explain this paradox, it is essential to understand the mechanism of protective immunity to these infectious agents and the nature of the immune defects caused by HIV itself.

The immune response to infectious agents

When an infectious agent invades the body, the immune system activates innate and acquired (adaptive) immune responses (Figure 6.1). Innate immune responses are not antigen-specific, do not 'mature' upon repeated exposure, and require no 'education'. They constitute the first line of immune defence and involve humoral

New and Resurgent Infections: Prediction, Detection and Management of Tomorrow's Epidemics.
Edited by B. Greenwood and K. De Cock.

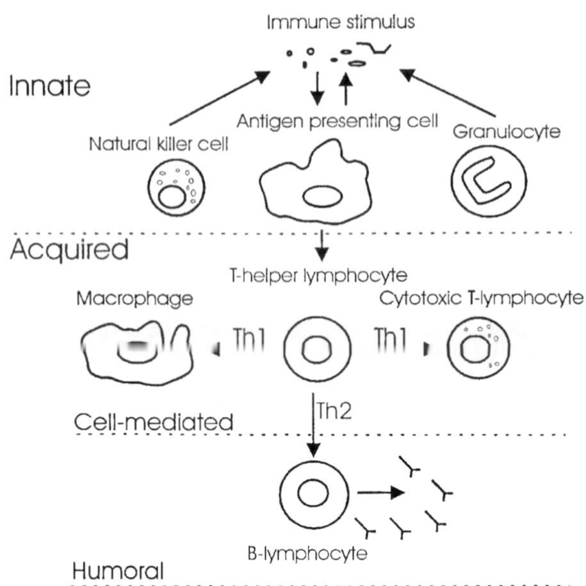

Figure 6.1 Immune responses to infectious agents comprise innate or non-specific responses and acquired or antigen-specific responses. The type of immune response is determined primarily by the nature of the infectious agent. Obligate intracellular viruses and parasites induce a cell-mediated immune response which is facilitated by cytokines which enhance cell-mediated immunity (Th-1 cytokines). Extracellular bacteria and parasites are neutralized mainly by a humoral immune response (antibodies, complement, etc.) which is driven by cytokines which enhance humoral immune responses (Th-2 cytokines)

components such as complement proteins, acute-phase proteins and other inflammatory mediators such as interferons and interleukins, as well as cellular components such as neutrophils, platelets, various tissue cells, mononuclear phagocytes and natural killer cells. On the other hand, adaptive immune responses are highly specific for a particular pathogen and improve with each re-exposure to the same pathogen. The adaptive immune response 'learns' and 'remembers' the infectious agent and can often prevent it from causing disease on a subsequent encounter. Cells which are central to adaptive immune responses are T-lymphocytes (T-cells) and B-lymphocytes (B-cells). B-cells produce antibodies whereas T-cells have another range of activities. Some subsets of T-cells are involved in helping B-cells to produce antibodies directed against extracellular pathogens (T-cell-dependent antibody production) whereas others interact with phagocytic and cytolytic cells and instruct them to destroy intracellular pathogens. Adaptive immune responses are generated in the context of the major histocompatibility complex (MHC) and are thus dependent on the genetic constitution of the host.

Mechanisms of protective immunity depend largely upon the nature of the infectious agents. Viruses are obligate intracellular organisms and require different immune responses than extracellular bacteria and parasites. As a rule, humoral immune responses are very efficient in neutralizing extracellular microbes whereas virus-infected cells and intracellular parasites can be destroyed only by cytolytic effector cells.

Host susceptibility or resistance to infection is determined, at least partially, by the type of immune response that the host develops. For instance, protective immune responses to intracellular viruses, bacteria and parasites such as cytomegalovirus, influenza virus, *Listeria monocytogenes*, *Mycobacterium leprae*, *M. tuberculosis*, *Leishmania* spp. and *Trypanosoma cruzi* are achieved predominantly through an adaptive cell-mediated immune response (Th1), whereas susceptibility to some of these agents is seen in individuals who mount a predominantly humoral immune (Th2) response.

Environmental factors can selectively interfere with either one or with both arms of the immune response and thus change the host susceptibility to infectious agents. Host factors which influence the immune response include genetic determinants and age. Environmental factors that can modulate the immune response include malnutrition, immunosuppressants, co-infections, mental stress, depression and exposure to pollutants and immunotoxins (Table 6.1).

Effect of the nutritional status on the immune response

Nutritional status is a well recognized determinant of immunocompetence. Nutritional disorders, affecting several hundred million people worldwide, can increase morbidity and mortality from many infections (Chandra and Newberne, 1977). Among the factors that determine nutritional status are food quality, food quantity and digestive efficiency. In addition, infection itself can deprive the body of nutrients and contribute to immunodeficiency, thus establishing a vicious circle (Storey, 1993). At one end of the spectrum of malnutrition are the gross changes seen in protein-energy malnutrition (PEM). More subtle changes are observed when specific nutrients like certain minerals and trace elements are selectively lacking.

Several components of the immune system are impaired in children who suffer from severe malnutrition. In PEM, the observed immunological defects are partially due to the effect of malnutrition on the lymphoid tissues, which are particularly susceptible as a result of their rapid rate of turnover and synthesis of immunomodulating proteins. Thymus, spleen, lymph nodes and Peyer's patches are altered in size and structure in children with severe PEM (Chandra, 1992).

Skin test responses to recall-antigens (delayed hypersensitivity skin responses), a useful *in vivo* measure of cell-mediated immunity, are reduced. Complete anergy (non-responsiveness) to a battery of different antigens is sometimes seen. A profound reduction of CD4+ T-helper cells is found in PEM, resulting in a

Table 6.1 Environmental factors which can affect the immune response

Environmental factor	Immunological impairment	Mechanism	Further reading
Malnutrition			
Protein energy malnutrition (PEM)	IFN-γ and IL-2 production, phagocytic activity, complement pathway, mucosal IgA response, DTH, T-LPR	Atrophy of lymphoid organs	Chandra, 1992; Chandra and Kumar, 1994 (overview)
Trace element deficiency			
Fe, Zn, Cu, Se	T-LPR (mitogens), NK, CTL, intracellular killing of bacteria by phagocytes, lymphokine production, neutrophil function	Reduced antioxidant function (metalloenzymes catalase (Fe), superoxide dismutase (Zn/Cu), glutathione peroxidase (Se))	Good and Lorenz, 1992; Bendich, 1993; Weiss *et al*, 1995; Harbige, 1996
Vitamin deficiency			
Vitamin A	CMI, T-cell-dependent antibody production, secretory IgA production	Unknown	Rumore, 1993
Vitamin B6 and B12	DTH, T-LPR, CTL	Thymic atrophy, B6 and B12 mediate DNA synthesis	Miller, 1992 (overview)
Vitamin C, Vitamin E	DTH, T-LPR, neutrophil bactericidal function, mucosal surface integrity	Antioxidant, co-factor in hydroxylation of proline and lysine (collagen synthesis)	Harbige, 1996; Chew, 1995
Neurological stress			
Mental stress	NK, CTL	(?) Neuropeptide receptors on immune cells	Cohen, 1995; Cohen and Herbert, 1996; Glaser *et al*, 1992; Irwin, 1988; Maes *et al*, 1991
Severe depression	NK, T-LPR		

Immune suppressants			
Azathioprine	CMI and humoral immunity (blocks DNA synthesis)	Interferes with purine biosynthesis	Sigal and Dumont, 1993 (overview)
Steroids	CMI, IFN-γ-antagonist, anti-inflammatory molecule	Steroid receptor on immune cells	Lew *et al*, 1988
Cyclosporin, FK-506	CMI (blocks lymphocyte activation)	Blocks IL-2 gene transcription	Sigal and Dumont, 1992
Rapamycin	CMI (blocks lymphocyte activation)	Blocks intracellular signalling through IL-2-R?	Sigal and Dumont, 1992
Environmental pollution			
Pesticides			
PCDDs, PCBs, PCDFs	NK, T-LPR, DTH, MLR, primary antigen-specific responses	TCDD binding to a cytosolic protein, the aryl hydrocarbon (*Ah*-) receptor, resemblance to TCDDs	de Swart *et al*, 1994, 1995; Ross *et al*, 1995
Ultraviolet B radiation (stratospheric ozone depletion)	DTH responses in the skin	Impairs function of antigen-presenting cells of the skin (Langerhans cells)	Morison, 1989; Patz *et al*, 1996

CMI = cell-mediated immunity; NK = natural killer cells; CTL = cytotoxic T-lymphocytes; DTH = delayed type hypersensitivity; MLR = mixed lymphocyte reaction; T-LPR = T-lymphocyte proliferative responses; PCDDs = polychlorinated dibenzo-*p*-dioxins; TCDDs = 2,3,7,8-tetrachloro-dibenzo-*p*-dioxin; PCBs = polychlorinated biphenyls; PCDFs = polychlorinated dibenzofurans significant reduction of T-helper (Th1) activity which explains, to a large extent, the alteration of cellular functions seen in children with PEM. Humoral (Th2) responses are less affected, as shown by near normal serum antibody responses after immunisation with common antigens. Nevertheless, mucosal IgA responses can be seriously depressed, enhancing the risk of mucosal infections (Chandra and Kumari, 1994), which, by resulting in diarrhoea, can further aggravate nutritional status and hence immune competence.

Some minerals, such as potassium, sodium, calcium, phosphorus and magnesium, are present in large amounts in the body. Others, such as selenium, zinc, iron and copper, are required only in small quantities, but nutritional deficiency of those trace elements can occur if available food lacks diversity. Enzyme and metabolic function may be significantly reduced by deficiencies in trace elements and vitamins. The most thoroughly studied trace element and vitamin deficiencies are those involving zinc, copper, iron, selenium, and vitamins A, B and E. Iron deficiency is the most common single nutrient deficiency, occurring in both developed and underdeveloped countries. It is characterized by reduced intracellular killing of bacteria by phagocytes, decreased T-cell numbers, reduced lymphocyte transformation to mitogens and by lowered lymphokine production (Weiss *et al*, 1995). The cellular basis of these various effects is reduced activity of ribonucleotidyl reductase (explaining the decreased proliferative responses depending on DNA and RNA synthesis) and decreased myeloperoxidase activity and hydroxyl radical production (explaining the deficient intracellular killing of bacteria by phagocytes). Zinc deficiency is associated with a depressed antibody production to heterologous antigens, reduced lymphocyte proliferative responses to mitogens, and depressed polymorphonuclear neutrophil, natural killer and cytotoxic T-cell function (Good and Lorenz, 1992). Selenium is necessary in sufficient amounts for protective immune responses to viruses. A critically low selenium level impairs T-cell functions and decreases natural killer cell activity (Harbige, 1996). Zinc, copper and iron are important in the antioxidant activity of some metallo-enzymes which neutralise intracellular free radicals. Free radicals and reactive oxygen species are produced by immune cells to destroy invading pathogens whereas the antioxidative system ensures that the formation of free radicals in living cells does not result in cellular damage (Bendich, 1993).

Deficiency of certain vitamins can also adversely affect immune functions. Vitamin A deficiency depresses cell-mediated immunity and T-cell-dependent antibody production, including secretory IgA production essential for the establishment of immunity to mucosal pathogens (Rumore, 1993). Vitamin E and C are naturally occurring antioxidant nutrients and enhance immunity, at least in part, by maintaining the functional and structural integrity of important immune cells (Chew, 1995; Harbige, 1996).

Immunosuppressants and susceptibility to infection

Immunosuppressants can increase the risk of infection significantly. Immunosuppressive agents can be grouped into several categories. Traditional immunosuppressives interfere with cellular metabolism and have a significant toxic effect. Examples of such antiproliferative agents are cyclophosphamide, methotrexate and azathioprine. They can cause non-specific suppression of both humoral and cell-mediated immune responses. Glucocorticosteroids suppress immune and inflammatory responses by inhibiting the expression of inflammatory mediators such as arachidonic acid metabolites and IL-1 (Lew *et al*, 1988). Another large group of agents inhibit signal transduction events at the cell surface or within the cell, resulting in non-specific immunosuppression and increased susceptibility to infection, although this is less drastic than that caused by the antiproliferative agents. Well known examples include cyclosporin A, FK-506 and rapamycin. They act as inhibitors of T-cell activation and interfere with the regulation of IL-2 gene transcription (CsA, FK506) or IL-2 receptor signal transduction (rapamycin) (Sigal and Dumont, 1992).

Mental stress, clinical depression and the immune system

Many studies have examined the relationship between mental stress, clinical depression and immunity (Cohen and Herbert, 1996). Emotional stress is often followed by increased susceptibility to bacterial and viral infections, at least for the less serious infectious diseases such as colds, influenza and herpes virus infection (Kiecolt-Glaser and Glaser, 1991; Cohen, 1995). The ability of mental stress to influence an immune response to a primary antigen has been well illustrated in a study of a group of students who were given a recombinant hepatitis B vaccine during a three-day academic examination period (Glaser *et al*, 1992). Those students who seroconverted after the first injection were significantly less stressed and anxious at the time of vaccination than those who did not seroconvert. Stress-associated reductions of important immunological anti-viral responses, such as those involving cytotoxic T-lymphocytes and natural killer cells, have also been observed in asymptomatic HIV-infected subjects (Evans *et al*, 1995). Similar observations were made in patients with severe depression (Irwin, 1988; Maes *et al*, 1991). Apparently, the immune system can be affected directly by innervation or by a neuro-endocrine cascade and vice versa. This bidirectional communication between the immune system and the central nervous system is achieved by means of common receptors and biologically active substances such as cytokines and neuropeptides (Savino and Dardenne, 1995).

Effect of environmental pollutants on the immune system

Because of the wide use of pesticides for domestic and industrial purposes, their potential immunotoxic effects are a matter of major concern for public health. Evidence that pesticides can severely impair immune functions in humans is scarce. Contact hypersensitivity is a well defined, although rare, consequence of exposure to pesticides, but immunologically mediated systemic reactions have been described only as debatable case reports (Vial *et al*, 1996). Studies in laboratory animals have shown that the mammalian immune system can be affected adversely by a variety of chemical agents (Vos and Luster, 1989; Saboori and Newcombe, 1992; Luster and Rosenthal, 1993; Lai *et al*, 1994) but, in most cases, these studies focused on acute immunotoxicity caused by relatively high levels of exposure. Potentially immunotoxic chemicals such as polychlorinated biphenyls (PCBs) and polychlorinated dibenzo-*p*-dioxins (PCDDs), dibenzofurans (PCDFs), hexachlorobenzene (HCB), dieldrin, β-hexachloro-cyclohexane (β-HCH) and dichlorodiphenyl trichloro-ethane (DDT) are present in abundance in the marine environment. Top predators are known to accumulate high levels of some of these xenobiotics. When morbillivirus infections led to massive mortalities among harbour seals in Europe in the early 1990s, it was speculated that this was caused by the adverse effect of environmental chemicals on the immune system of these animals. In a recent study carried out by de Swart *et al* (1995), statistically significant changes in cellular immune responses were detected in harbour seals that were fed on environmentally contaminated herring from the Baltic Sea. Whether induced immunological changes were the major determinant that promoted the virus infection and caused mass mortalities among seals is difficult to prove.

The mechanism of immune suppression induced by the most extensively studied group of immunotoxic chemicals, TCDD and related compounds including PCDDs, PCDFs and PCBs, is thought to be mediated by binding to a cytosolic protein, the aryl hydrocarbon receptor (Holsapple *et al*, 1991). The toxicity of these chemicals is largely dependent on their stereochemical resemblance to TCDD, the chemical with the highest affinity for this receptor. Through their interaction with this receptor, they can activate key protein kinases that are involved in the growth factor signal-transduction pathway (Matsumura, 1995).

Climatic factors can influence susceptibility to infectious diseases as well. Ultraviolet radiation is a possible factor involved in climate-related immune dysfunction. Ultraviolet B radiation induces selective biological alterations in the skin, including suppression of normal immune responses, probably through its effect on Langerhans cells, the most important antigen-presenting cells of the skin (Morison, 1989). The pathogenic consequences of UVB radiation can be observed in the exacerbation of infectious diseases and development of skin cancer (Vermeer and Hurks, 1994). UV-mediated immune suppression may become more important in the future as a consequence of an increased flux of ultraviolet radiation (Patz *et al*, 1996).

Susceptibility to HIV and the effect of HIV on the immune system

Cellular immune responses to HIV and disease progression

Human immune deficiency virus (HIV) is characterized by its dramatic effect on the immune system. It infects and kills CD4+ T-helper lymphocytes, which play a pivotal role in the generation of an immune response (Figure 6.1). Once an individual becomes infected with HIV, the host reacts with a vigorous immune response against the virus. HIV-specific cytotoxic T-cells are generated, killing infected cells, and neutralizing antibodies are produced which limit the spread of cell-free virus. Nevertheless, the virus escapes from these vigorous but apparently inadequate immune responses, resulting in a chronically overactivated immune system which finally collapses and leaves the host in a state of severe acquired immune deficiency (AIDS). Lymph nodes are the main reservoir for HIV, and even during the asymptomatic stage of the infection billions of virus particles are produced every day and millions of CD4+ T-cells are destroyed (Fauci *et al*, 1993; Ho *et al*, 1995; Wei *et al*, 1995).

CD8+ T-cells are thought to play an important role in the immune defence against HIV. Large numbers of activated cytotoxic CD8+ T-cells (CTL) are generated early after infection and may slow down disease progression (reviewed by Autran *et al*, 1996). Nevertheless, the persistence of virus replication indicates the inability of CTL to eradicate HIV. Moreover, during the asymptomatic stage of the infection, vigorous polyclonal CTL responses directed against HIV are associated with the generation of a large number of virus variants (Ho *et al*, 1995; Wei *et al*, 1995) which are no longer recognised by CTL (Phillips *et al*, 1991; Haas *et al*, 1996) and which ultimately result in disease progression.

CD8+ T-cells are also able to control HIV replication without killing infected cells. This antiviral activity appears to be mediated by soluble factors such as chemokines (Cocchi *et al*, 1995) and CD8+ T-cell antiviral factor (CAF) (reviewed by Levy *et al*, 1996). CD8+ T-cells from asymptomatic HIV-infected subjects produce high levels of these suppressor factors and it has been suggested that they are important in preventing progression to clinical disease (Levy *et al*, 1996).

CD8+ T-cells are activated by Th1-like cytokines (IL-2, IFN-γ, TNF-α) whereas Th2-like cytokines (IL-4, IL-5, IL-6, IL-10, IL-13) tend to suppress cell-mediated immune responses. Studies have suggested that HIV disease progression is associated with a profound shift from a 'protective' cell-mediated (Th1) to a 'non-protective' humoral (Th2) immune response (Clerici and Shearer, 1993) but this hypothesis has generated a great deal of controversy due to discordant findings from different laboratories and is not accepted universally.

Susceptibility or resistance to infection with HIV

During the past five years, it has become clear that (i) a small group of HIV-seropositive individuals who have been infected for at least 10 years have not progressed to AIDS (so-called long-term non-progressors or LTNP) and (ii) there exists a small group of HIV-seronegative individuals who have been exposed to the virus many times and yet have not seroconverted or become infected.

The majority of LTNP have high levels of HIV-specific CTL in their peripheral blood and in their lymph nodes (Pantaleo *et al*, 1995) and their CD8+ T-lymphocytes produce large quantities of HIV suppressor factor (Levy *et al*, 1996) responses that are thought to play an important role in preventing HIV disease progression in LTNP.

Interestingly, HIV-specific cellular immune responses have been detected in HIV seronegative individuals who have been exposed to the virus many times without being infected, suggesting that innate and/or naturally acquired immune responses to HIV may be protective in rare individuals (reviewed by Shearer and Clerici, 1996). Peripheral blood mononuclear cells obtained from different individuals are not equally permissive to HIV, and CD4+ T-cells taken from apparently HIV-'resistant' subjects produce more chemokines (RANTES, MIP-1 and MIP-1β) than do CD4+ T-cells obtained from HIV-susceptible individuals (Paxton *et al*, 1996). Although it had already been shown that these chemokines could prevent infection of monocytes by monocytotropic HIV strains (Cocchi *et al*, 1995), the precise mechanism remained unknown until the discovery of the HIV co-receptors. The CD4 molecule, which is expressed at the cell surface of helper T-cells and monocytes, was identified as the primary cell receptor for HIV many years ago and, although HIV binds tightly to CD4, expression of CD4 was found to be insufficient to allow HIV entry into non-human cells (Maddon *et al*, 1986). The discovery that the chemokine receptor CCR5 acts as a co-receptor for HIV (Alkhatib *et al*, 1996) explains why and how certain chemokines can block HIV infection. They interfere with HIV infection by binding to and blocking receptor availability to HIV. Another member of the chemokine-receptor family, CXCR4 (fusin), had already been identified earlier as a co-receptor for lymphotropic HIV variants (Feng *et al*, 1996).

Shortly after the discovery of the two co-receptors for HIV, Samson *et al* (1996), Dean *et al* (1996) and Liu *et al* (1996) described a polymorphism in the gene coding for CCR5. The presence of a mutation in this gene, a 32 base pair deletion, confers resistance or partial resistance to HIV infection. The gene product results in a non-functional receptor that does not support membrane fusion of HIV with its target cell. Population studies indicate that the homozygous defect is found in 1–2% of Caucasians, and the heterozygous defect in 13–16% of this population (Samson *et al*, 1996; Huang *et al*, 1996). So far, no HIV-infected Caucasians, homozygous for the mutation, have been found. Whether heterozygotes are also less susceptible to HIV infection is still controversial (Samson *et al*, 1996; Huang *et al*, 1996). This protective allele appears to be absent in black populations from Western and Central Africa and from populations in Japan (Samson *et al*, 1996; Huang *et al*, 1996). Since apparent resistance to HIV has also been observed in these populations (Fowke *et al*, 1996), factors other than defective co-receptors must also be involved.

Environmental factors can affect susceptibility to HIV infection

Successful replication of HIV in CD4+ T-lymphocytes is determined by the state of activation of HIV-infected cells. Only activated cells produce large amounts of infectious virus particles. Therefore, concurrent infections, which stimulate the immune system, may enhance HIV replication in infected cells and accelerate HIV disease progression. In addition, infections may activate the immune system of HIV-seronegative subjects and render them more susceptible to infection with HIV. As a consequence, one might expect to find a higher susceptibility to HIV in areas where many other infectious diseases are prevalent, such as most developing countries. The rapid spread of HIV in developing countries may, in part, be accounted for by this phenomenon. Infections, such as tuberculosis (TB), that chronically activate the immune system could be especially damaging (Vanham *et al*, 1996). *Mycobacterium tuberculosis* (MTB) can activate the expression of HIV in latently infected monocytic cell lines, and monocytes obtained from TB patients support HIV replication better than monocytes from control persons (Toossi *et al*, 1993; Lederman *et al*, 1994). MTB increases HIV replication in peripheral blood mononuclear cells and this is correlated with the level of cellular activation which is a predominant characteristic of HIV-infected subjects (Kestens *et al*, 1992; 1994; Goletti *et al*, 1996). HIV replication was found to increase 5- to 160-fold during the acute phase of MTB disease (Goletti *et al*, 1996). These observations provide the underlying explanation for the clinical finding that infection with MTB can accelerate the clinical course of HIV (Whalen *et al*, 1995).

Both ulcerative and non-ulcerative sexually transmitted diseases (STDs) are known to increase susceptibility to HIV (Laga *et al*, 1993; Torian *et al*, 1995). Ulcerative STDs probably facilitate HIV entry through mucosal lesions, rather than by their effect on the immune system. The precise role of non-ulcerative STDs, such as gonorrhoeal, chlamydial and trichomonal infections, needs further elucidation.

Infections such as those caused by *Schistosoma mansoni* infection may drive the immune response towards a Th2-like profile and increase susceptibility to HIV infection. In mice infected with *S. mansoni*, suppression of Th1 reactivity by a dominant Th2 response has been shown to result in failure of virus-specific CD8+ T-cell responses to vaccinia virus (Actor *et al*, 1993). This suggests that helminth infections can influence immune responses to concurrent viral infections (Kullberg *et al*, 1992). Bentwich *et al* (1996) have shown a very high prevalence of helminthic and other infections associated with extreme immune dysregulation as well as a high prevalence of HIV-1 in Ethiopian immigrants to Israel. Although one of the striking characteristics of the AIDS epidemic in Africa is the way the disease differs from the pattern seen in other areas, the reasons for this are not clear. It has been suggested that changes in the host immune response caused by endemic infections and mostly helminth infections could account for at least a part of this pattern (Bentwich *et al*, 1995).

Immunisation of HIV-seropositive patients with recall antigens temporarily enhances HIV replication in infected subjects (Stanley *et al*, 1996), raising the question of the advisability of vaccinations in HIV-infected subjects. However, the protection afforded in most cases by vaccination outweighs the potential risks from a transient increase in immune activation.

HIV changes the susceptibility to other infectious diseases

HIV induces progressive and selective immune defects in infected humans. Cell-mediated immune responses of the Th1 type which are required to confer protective immunity against pathogens are particularly compromised. Epidemiological data have demonstrated that HIV-infected individuals are more susceptible to MTB and that the HIV epidemic has a central role in the worldwide resurgence of this infection (Barnes *et al*, 1991). A study conducted by Burwen *et al* (1995) estimated that HIV-induced immunosuppression accounts for a minimum of 30% of the excess TB cases during the period 1985–1990 in the US. In Côte d'Ivoire, the incidence of tuberculosis was 1104 per 100 000 among HIV-infected persons in 1991 but only 96 per 100 000 in HIV-seronegative persons, a figure which is lower than the overall incidence measured in 1981 (155 per 100 000) (Richards *et al*, 1995). HIV affects not only the incidence of MTB but also its clinical presentation. Reactivation of pulmonary TB may occur early in HIV infection whereas extrapulmonary or atypical disease is seen in patients with profound HIV-induced immunodeficiency (Lucas and Nelson, 1994).

Visceral leishmaniasis (*Leishmania donovani*) is another opportunistic infection seen with increased frequency in patients infected with HIV who live in areas endemic for Leishmania. As a result of HIV, visceral leishmaniasis is becoming more important in non-endemic areas as well (Albrecht *et al*, 1996).

Toxoplasmosis, *Pneumocystis carinii* and *Herpes simplex* are classical examples of latent infections which can be reactivated by HIV. In contrast, leprosy (*M. leprae*), malaria (*Plasmodium falciparum*) and amoebiasis (*Entamoeba histolytica*), which are at least partially controlled by cell-mediated immunity and which should theoretically be more frequent in HIV-positive people than in HIV-negatives, do not appear to be more frequent or more aggressive in HIV-infected subjects. The reasons for this are unclear.

Conclusion

It is clear that a variety of environmental factors can disturb the integrity of the immune system in a direct or indirect manner. They can change the susceptibility of the host to infection and they may have a role in the spread of new or resurgent infectious diseases. Numerous publications have demonstrated that many of these factors induce measurable changes in cellular and humoral immunity. The relative increase in susceptibility to infection depends on the nature of the infectious agent and on the type and degree of immune perturbation.

Acknowledgements

The authors thank Ms Greet Verhulst for secretarial assistance.

References

Actor JK, Shirai M, Kullberg MC, Buller RM, Sher A, Berzofsky JA. Helminth infection results in decreased virus-specific CD8+ cytotoxic T-cell and Th1-cytokine responses as well as delayed virus clearance. *Proceedings of the National Academy of Sciences of the USA*, 1993; **90**: 948–952

Akhatib G, Combadiere C, Broder CC *et al.* CC CKRS: a RANTES, MIP-1 alpha, MIP-1 beta receptor as a fusion cofactor for macrophage-tropic HIV-1. *Science*, 1996; **272**: 1955–1958

Albrecht H, Sobottka I, Emminger C *et al.* Visceral leishmaniasis emerging as an important opportunistic infection in HIV-infected persons living in areas nonendemic for *Leishmania donovani. Archives of Pathology and Laboratory Medicine*, 1996; **120**: 189–198

Autran B, Hadida F, Haas G. Evolution and plasticity of CTL responses against HIV. *Current Opinions in Immunology*, 1996; **8**: 546–553

Barnes PF, Bloch AB, Davidson PT, Snider DE. Tuberculosis in patients with human immunodeficiency virus infection. *New England Journal of Medicine*, 1991; **324**: 1644–1650

Bendich A. Physiological role of antioxidants in the immune system. *Journal of Dairy Sciences*, 1993; **76**: 2789–2794

Bentwich Z, Kalinkovich A, Weisman Z. Immune activation is a dominant factor in the pathogenesis of African AIDS. *Immunology Today*, 1995; **16**: 187–191

Bentwich Z, Weisman Z, Moroz C, Bar-Yehuda S, Kalinkovich A. Immune dysregulation in Ethiopian immigrants in Israel: Relevance to helminth infections? *Clinical and Experimental Immunology*, 1996; **103**: 239–243

Burwen DR, Bloch AB, Griffin LD, Ciesielski CA, Stern HA, Onorato IM. National trends in the concurrence of tuberculosis and acquired immunodeficiency syndrome. *Archives of Internal Medicine*, 1995; **155**: 1281–1286

Chandra RK. Nutrition and immunoregulation. Significance for host resistance to tumors and infectious diseases in humans and rodents. *Journal of Nutrition*, 1992; **122**: 754–757

Chandra RK, Kumari S. Nutrition and immunity: an overview. *Journal of Nutrition*, 1994; **124 (8 Suppl.)**: 1433S–1435S

Chandra RK, Newberne PM (eds). *Nutrition, Immunity and Infection: Mechanisms of Interactions*. New York: Plenum Press, 1977

Chew BP. Antioxidant vitamins affect food animal immunity and health. *Journal of Nutrition*, 1995; **125 (6 Suppl.)**: 1804S–1808S

Clerici M, Shearer GM. A Th1-Th2 switch is a critical step in the etiology of HIV infection. *Immunology Today*, 1993; **14**: 107–111

Cocchi F, Devico AL, Garzino-Demo A, Arya SK, Gallo RC, Lusso P. Identification of RANTES, MIP-1 alpha, and MIP-1 beta as the major HIV-suppressive factors produced by CD8(+) T cells. *Science*, 1995; **270**: 1811–1815

Cohen S. Psychological stress and susceptibility to upper respiratory infections. *American Journal of Respiratory and Critical Care Medicine*, 1995; **152**: S53–S58

Cohen S, Herbert TB. Health psychology: psychological factors and physical disease from the perspective of human psychoneuroimmunology. *Annual Review of Psychology*, 1996; **47**: 113–142

de Swart RL, Ross PS, Vedder LJ *et al.* Impairment of immune function in harbor seals (*Phoca vitulina*) feeding on fish from polluted waters. *Ambio*, 1994; **23**: 155–159

de Swart RL, Ross PS, Timmerman HH *et al.* Impaired cellular immune response in harbour seals (*Phoca vitulina*) feeding on environmentally contaminated herring. *Clinical and Experimental Immunology*, 1995; **101**: 480–486

Dean M, Carrington M, Winkler C *et al.* Genetic restriction of HIV-1 infection and progression to AIDS by a deletion allele of the CKR5 structural gene. Hemophilia Growth and Development Study, Multicenter AIDS Cohort Study, Multicenter Hemophilia Cohort Study, San Francisco City Cohort ALIVE Study. *Science*, 1996; **273**: 1856–1862

Evans DL, Leserman J, Perkins DO *et al.* Stress-associated reductions of cytotoxic T lymphocytes and natural killer cells in asymptomatic HIV infection. *American Journal of Psychiatry*, 1995; **152**: 543–550

Fauci AS, Pantaleo G, Embretson J, Haase AT. Viral burden and HIV disease—reply. *Nature*, 1993; **364**: 291–292

Feng Y, Broder CC, Kennedy PE, Berger EA. HIV-1 entry cofactor: functional cDNA cloning of a seven-transmembrane, G protein-coupled receptor. *Science*, 1996; **272**: 872–877

Fowke KR, Nagelkerke NJD, Kimani J *et al.* Resistance to HIV-1 infection among persistently seronegative prostitutes in Nairobi, Kenya. *Lancet*, 1996; **348**: 1347–1351

Glaser R, Kiecolt-Glaser JK, Bonneau RH, Malarkey W, Kennedy S, Hughes J. Stress-induced modulation of the immune response to recombinant hepatitis-B vaccine. *Psychosomatic Medicine*, 1992; **54**: 22–29

Goletti D, Weissman D, Jackson RW *et al.* Effect of *Mycobacterium tuberculosis* on HIV replication. Role of immune activation. *Journal of Immunology*, 1996; **157**: 1271–1278

Good RA, Lorenz E. Nutrition and cellular immunity. *International Journal of Immunopharmacology*, 1992; **14**: 361–366

Haas G, Plikat U, Debre P *et al.* Dynamics of viral variants in HIV-I Nef and specific cytotoxic T lymphocytes in vivo. *Journal of Immunology*, 1996; **157**: 4212–4221

Harbige LS. Nutrition and immunity with emphasis on infection and autoimmune disease. *Nutrition and Health*, 1996; **10**: 285–312

Ho DD, Neumann AU, Perelson AS, Chen W, Leonard JM, Markowitz M. Rapid turnover of plasma virions and CD4 lymphocytes in HIV-1 infection. *Nature*, 1995; **373**: 123–126

Holsapple MP, Morris DL, Wood SC, Snyder NK. 2,3,7,8-tetrachlorodibenzo-p-dioxin-induced changes in immunocompetence: possible mechanisms. *Annual Review of Pharmacology and Toxicology*, 1991; **31**: 73–100

Huang Y, Paxton WA, Wolinsky SM *et al.* The role of a mutant CCR5 allele in HIV-1 transmission and disease progression. *Nature Medicine*, 1996; **2**: 1240–1243

Irwin M. Depression and immune function. *Stress Medicine*, 1988; **14**: 95–103

Kestens L, Vanham G, Gigase P *et al.* Expression of activation antigens, HLA-DR and CD38 on CD8 lymphocytes during HIV-1 infection. *AIDS*, 1992; **6**: 793–797

Kestens L, Vanham G, Vereecken C *et al.* Selective increase of activation antigens HLA-DR and CD38 on CD4(+)CD45RO(+) T lymphocytes during HIV-1 infection. *Clinical and Experimental Immunology*, 1994; **95**: 436–441

Kiecolt-Glaser JK, Glaser R. Stress and immune function in humans. In: Ader R, Felten

DL,Cohen N (eds), *Psychoneuroimmunology*. San Diego, CA: Academic Press, 1991, pp 849–867

Kullberg MC, Pearce EJ, Hieny SE, Sher A, Berzofsky JA. Infection with *Schistosoma mansoni* alters Th1-Th2 cytokine responses to a non-parasite antigen. *Journal of Immunology*, 1992; **148**: 3264–3270

Laga M, Manoka A, Kivuvu M *et al.* Non-ulcerative sexually transmitted diseases as risk factors for HIV-1 transmission in women: results from a cohort study. *AIDS*, 1993; **7**: 95–102

Lai ZW, Kremer J, Gleichmann E, Esser C. 3,3′,4,4′-tetrachlorobiphenyl (TCB) inhibits proliferation of immature thymocytes in fetal thymus organ culture. *Scandinavian Journal of Immunology*, 1994; **39**: 480–488

Lederman MM, Georges DL, Kusner DJ, Mudido P, Giam CZ, Toossi Z. *Mycobacterium tuberculosis* and its purified protein derivative activate expression of the human immunodeficiency virus. *Journal of Acquired Immune Deficiency Syndromes*, 1994; **7**: 727–733

Levy JA, Mackewicz CE, Barker E. Controlling HIV pathogenesis: the role of the noncytotoxic anti-HIV response of CD8(+) T cells. *Immunology Today*, 1996; **17**: 217–224

Lew W, Oppenheim JJ, Matsushima K. Analysis of the suppression of IL-1 alpha and IL-1 beta production in human peripheral blood mononuclear adherent cells by a glucocorticoid hormone. *Journal of Immunology*, 1988; **140**: 1895–1902

Liu R, Paxton WA, Choe S *et al.* Homozygous defect in HIV-1 coreceptor accounts for resistance of some multiply-exposed individuals to HIV-1 infection. *Cell*, 1996; **86**: 367–377

Lucas S, Nelson AM. Pathogenesis of tuberculosis in human immunodeficiency virus-infected people. In: Bloom BR (ed), *Tuberculosis: Pathogenesis, Protection and Control*. Washington, DC: American Society for Microbiology Press, 1994, pp 503–513

Luster MI, Rosenthal GJ. Chemical agents and the immune response. *Environmental Health Perspectives*, 1993; **100**: 219–236

Maddon PJ, Dalgleish AG, McDougal JS, Clapham PR, Weiss R, Axel R. The T4 gene encodes the AIDS virus receptor and is expressed in the immune system and the brain. *Cell*, 1986; **47**: 333–348

Maes M, Bosmans E, Suy E, Minner B, Raus J. A further exploration of the relationships between immune parameters and the HPA-axis activity in depressed patients. *Psychological Medicine*, 1991; **21**: 313–320

Matsumura F. Mechanism of action of dioxin-type chemicals, pesticides, and other xenobiotics affecting nutritional indexes. *American Journal of Clinical Nutrition*, 1995; **61**: 695S–701S

Miller LT. Vitamin B group and the immune system. In: Roit IM, Delves PJ (eds), *Encyclopedia of Immunology*. London: Academic Press, 1992, pp 1564–1565

Morison W. Effects of ultraviolet radiation on the immune system in humans. *Photochemistry and Photobiology*, 1989; **50**: 515–524

Pantaleo G, Menzo S, Vaccarezza M *et al.* Studies in subjects with long term nonprogressive human immunodeficiency virus infection. *New England Journal of Medicine*, 1995; **332**: 209–216

Patz JA, Epstein PR, Burke TA, Balbus JM. Global climate change and emerging infectious diseases. *Journal of the American Medical Association*, 1996; **275**: 217–223

Paxton WA, Martin SR, Tse D *et al.* Relative resistance to HIV-1 infection of CD4 lymphocytes from persons who remain uninfected despite multiple high-risk sexual exposures. *Nature Medicine*, 1996; **2**: 412–417

Phillips RE, Rowland-Jones S, Nixon DF *et al.* Human immunodeficiency virus genetic variation that can escape cytotoxic T-cell recognition. *Nature*, 1991; **354**: 453–459

Richards SB, St Louis ME, Nieburg P *et al.* Impact of the HIV epidemic on trends in tuberculosis in Abidjan, Côte d'Ivoire. *Tubercle and Lung Disease*, 1995; **76**: 11–16

Ross PS, de Swart RL, Reijnders PJ, Van Loveren H, Vos JG, Osterhaus AD. Contaminant-related suppression of delayed-type hypersensitivity and antibody responses in harbor seals fed herring from the Baltic Sea. *Environmental Health Perspectives*, 1995; **103**: 162–167

Rumore MM. Vitamin A as an immunomodulating agent. *Clinical Pharmacology and Therapeutics*, 1993; **12**: 506–514

Saboori AM, Newcombe DS. Environmental chemicals with immunotoxic properties. In: Newcombe DS, Rose NR, Bloom JC (eds), *Clinical Immunotoxicology*. New York: Raven Press, 1992, pp 365–400

Samson M, Libert F, Doranz BJ *et al.* Resistance to HIV-1 infection in Caucasian individuals bearing mutant alleles of the CCR-5 chemokine receptor gene. *Nature*, 1996; **382**: 722–725

Savino W, Dardenne M. Immune–neuroendocrine interactions. *Immunology Today*, 1995; **16**: 318–322

Shearer GM, Clerici M. Protective immunity against HIV infection: has nature done the experiment for us? *Immunology Today*, 1996; **17**: 21–24

Sigal NH, Dumont FJ. Cyclosporin A, FK-506 and rapamycin: pharmacologic probes of lymphocyte signal transduction. *Annual Review of Immunology*, 1992; **10**: 519–560

Sigal NH, Dumont FJ. Immunosuppression. In: Paul WE (ed), *Fundamental Immunology*. New York: Raven Press, 1993, pp 903–915

Stanley SK, Ostrowski MA, Justement JS *et al.* Effect of immunization with a common recall antigen on viral expression in patients infected with human immunodeficiency virus type 1. *New England Journal of Medicine*, 1996; **334**: 1222–1230

Storey DM. Filariasis: nutritional interactions in human and animal hosts. *Parasitology*, 1993; **107**: S147–S158

Toossi Z, Sierra-Madero JG, Blinkhorn RA, Mettler MA, Rich EA. Enhanced susceptibility of blood monocytes from patients with pulmonary tuberculosis to productive infection with human immunodeficiency virus type 1. *Journal of Experimental Medicine*, 1993; **177**: 1511–1516

Torian LV, Weisfuse IB, Makki HA, Benson DA, DiCamillo LM, Toribio FE. Increasing HIV-1 seroprevalence associated with genital ulcer disease, New York City, 1990–1992. *AIDS*, 1995; **9**: 177–181

Vanham G, Edmonds K, Qing L *et al.* Generalized immune activation in pulmonary tuberculosis: Co-activation with HIV infection. *Clinical and Experimental Immunology*, 1996; **103**: 30–34

Vermeer BJ, Hurks M. The clinical relevance of immunosuppression by UV irradiation. *Journal of Photochemistry and Photobiology–B, Biology*, 1994; **24**: 149–154

Vial T, Nicolas B, Descotes J. Clinical immunotoxicity of pesticides. *Journal of Toxicology and Environmental Health*, 1996; **48**: 215–229

Vos JG, Luster MI. Immune alterations. In: Kimbrough RD, Jensen S (eds), *Halogenated Biphenyls, Terphenyls, Naphthalenes, Dibenzodioxins and Related Products*. Amsterdam: Elsevier Science Publishers BV, 1989, pp 295–322

Wei X, Ghosh SK, Taylor ME *et al.* Viral dynamics in human immunodeficiency virus type 1 infection. *Nature*, 1995; **373**: 117–122

Weiss G, Wachter H, Fuchs D. Linkage of cell-mediated immunity to iron metabolism. *Immunology Today*, 1995; **16**: 495–500

Whalen C, Horsburgh CR, Hom D, Lahart C, Simberkoff M, Ellner J. Accelerated course of human immunodeficiency virus infection after tuberculosis. *American Journal of Respiratory and Critical Care Medicine*, 1995; **151**: 129–135

7
Malaria: the role of agriculture in changing the epidemiology of malaria

Melba Gomes, Kenneth Linthicum* and Mitiku Haile†

*Special Programme for Research and Training in Tropical Diseases, World Health Organization, Geneva, Switzerland, *Armed Forces Research Institute for Medicine, Bangkok, Thailand and †Mekelle University College, Mekelle, Ethiopia*

Malaria is the most important of the tropical diseases with which research directed by the World Health Organization's Special Programme for Research and Training in Tropical Diseases (TDR) is most intimately associated. The emergence and epidemic potential of this disease are often associated with a sudden increase in the degree of contact between host, vector and parasite. The critical link in this chain is the vector which, in the case of malaria, is the anopheles mosquito. Conditions which permit an explosion of the vector population and which retain its ability to transmit the pathogen to significant numbers of humans create the potential for an epidemic. Attempts to explain epidemics through a narrow focus on pathogen virulence may be misleading because they ignore the role that economic and social forces play in enhancing transmission potential.

Although many anopheline mosquitoes can carry and transmit the malaria parasite to humans, three species play a dominant role in the transmission of *Plasmodium falciparum* malaria, which can cause complicated malaria and death. Changes in the ecosystem which influence the habitat for *Anopheles dirus* in south-east Asia, *An. gambiae* in Africa and *An. darlingi* in Latin America, influence the potential for malaria transmission within these areas. These three mosquitoes are important because their behaviour and reproductive patterns allow them to be efficient disease transmitters. Moreover, their adaptability to variations in local habitat, for example, altitude, temperature, ambient humidity, rainfall patterns, shade, tree cover and soil composition, enhances their ability to survive most efforts to eliminate them.

New and Resurgent Infections: Prediction, Detection and Management of Tomorrow's Epidemics.
Edited by B. Greenwood and K. De Cock.

Recent assessments by WHO suggest that epidemic malaria may become more prevalent as a result in part of changes in land use brought about by development activities funded on compelling economic grounds. For example, agricultural or water development projects have important economic benefits but they can also generate serious adverse health outcomes such as an increase in the incidence of malaria, although such outcomes can be minimized or eliminated with advance information, better screening and project design. The complex interaction of events that can result in a heightened morbidity and mortality from malaria following changes in agricultural practice is illustrated in the following two case examples.

Case 1. Thailand: commercial tree crop plantations

Today Thailand has the highest level of multi-drug resistant malaria in the world. Chloroquine was used for the treatment of uncomplicated malaria, despite the detection of resistant strains in 1957, until the introduction of Fansidar (sulfadoxine/pyrimethamine) in 1973. This was followed by the introduction of mefloquine/sulfadoxine/pyramethamine (MSP) in 1985, mefloquine in 1990–91, quinine/tetracyline in 1993, and mefloquine/artesunate in 1994 for highly drug-resistant areas. The deployment of artesunate signifies the use of the last group of drugs which are effective in the treatment of uncomplicated malaria in peripheral health facilities. Although there is presently no known resistance to this group of compounds, there is a risk that increases in the prevalence of malaria within south-east Asia will result in the emergence of resistance to the artemisinin derivatives and thus lead to higher levels of malaria and higher death rates from malaria tomorrow. For this reason, the issue of whether and how increases in malaria transmission occur in south-east Asia is of global significance since any increase in transmission in the area may facilitate the emergence of more resistant parasite strains which are a threat to the world as a whole.

Why and how might there be an increase in the prevalence of malaria in south-east Asia? Is there any evidence within the region that malaria has returned from areas where it had supposedly been eliminated and is spreading to unaffected areas? Answering this question depends upon an intimate knowledge of the vector which transmits malaria in South-east Asia.

In the south-east Asian region, the primary vector for *P. falciparum* malaria is *An. dirus*. This is a mosquito whose natural habitat is deep forest. Historically, malaria in south-east Asia has been most stable and dangerous in areas where humans have lived in contact with natural tropical forests. The name 'dirus' means 'dangerous' and this species, which inhabits jungles from India to Vietnam and China, is a most efficient vector of human malaria. It is a large mosquito and part of its efficiency lies in the fact that it takes a large blood meal. A second factor is that it is relatively long-lived, a most important component in being able to transmit malaria. It prefers to lay its eggs in the shade which it can discern even in starlight.

Its density falls when the tree canopy is reduced, and this is the main reason why—in south-east Asia—if there are no trees, there is no *An. dirus* and, as a result, no malaria. Indeed, it has been suggested (Rosenberg *et al*, 1990) that the reduction in the incidence of malaria observed in the region has been achieved largely through reduction of forest cover, rather than through disease-specific control efforts!

In Thailand, the incidence of malaria is greatest in the provinces along the Burmese and Cambodian borders, where forest covers more than 35% of the area of the province. On the non-Thai side of the border, these areas are heavily forested and occupied by ethnic minorities. On the Thai side of the border, forests have been reduced, and outside the refugee camps the deforested areas are now being replanted for watershed protection and commercial revenue. Significant reductions in malaria incidence have been made by closing the border with Cambodia, which has discouraged illegal movements between the two countries for gem mining and logging activities. Nevertheless, malaria continues to persist in the region, even among groups who do not cross the borders (children and students), raising the question about the extent to which new tree plantations in formerly forested areas have led to reintroduction of malaria.

Methodology

Answering this question has required an in-depth analysis of changes in land use during the past 10 years, assessment of changes in land use which might have recreated a suitable habitat for *An. dirus*, and an examination of the transmission potential and incidence of malaria in new commercial tree crop plantations. This assessment was done using several satellite maps (1986, 1990, 1995) of areas chosen because of their persistent malaria endemicity despite rigorous control efforts (Linthicum *et al*, 1996), classification of the land use in these areas from satellite and land-use maps and attribution of malaria incidence by land-use category. The Land Satellite Thematic Mapper provided data which were examined using ERDAS image processing software to establish preliminary vegetation categories, later confirmed (for 1995) by ground truth observations. Existing land-use data for Chantaburi and Kanchanaburi Provinces were obtained from the Land Development Department, Ministry of Agriculture and Cooperatives for 1986 and 1991. These maps were digitised using ARC/Info GIS software, and the total area for each land-use type was calculated.

Malaria incidence data for 1985, 1989 and 1994 were obtained from the Malaria Control Division and placed in a GIS database. These maps were used to depict *P. falciparum* cases and the presumptive origin of the cases (within the district, outside the district, across the border).

Results

Figures 7.1, 7.2 and 7.3 show data on the changing incidence of malaria between 1991 and 1994 by province. They show the highest case incidence in Kanchanaburi

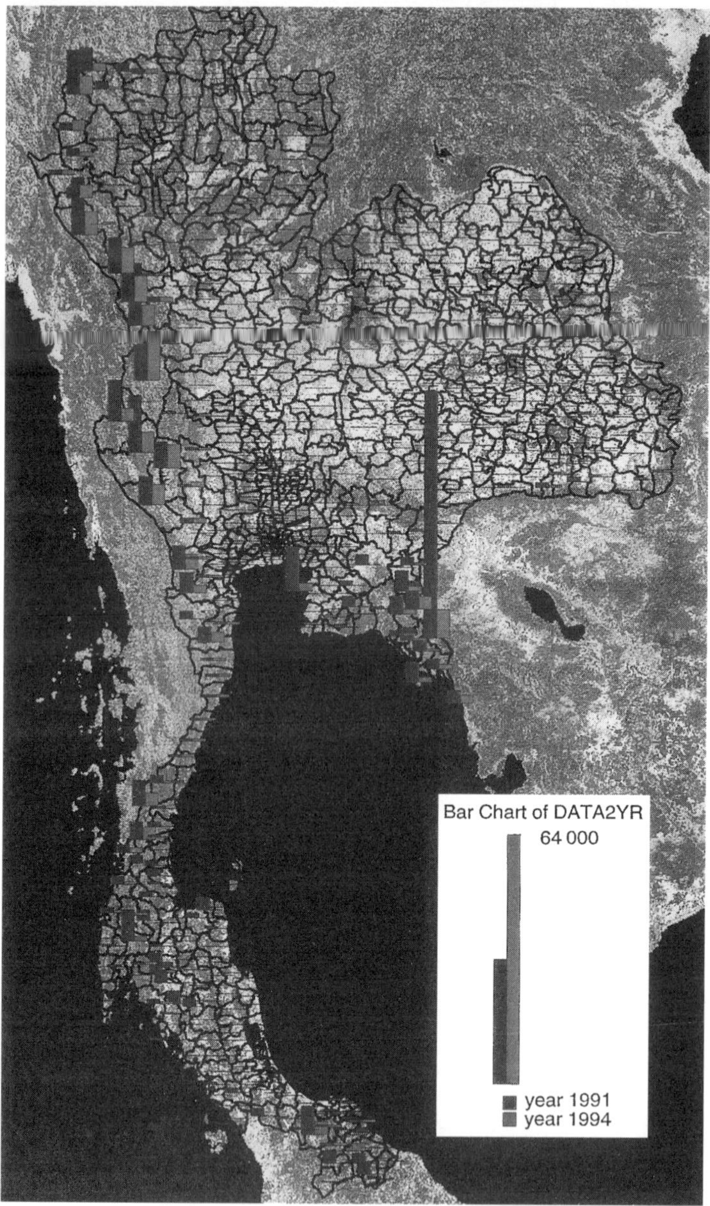

Figure 7.1 Malaria incidence in Thailand by district for 1991 and 1994. Malaria incidence is shown per 100 000 population of each district. Malaria incidence and district boundary data are displayed over a 1992–93 composite NOAA/NDVI image. This image has been given false colours to show areas with high green-leaf biomass as dark colour. In general when moving from dark to light decreasing vegetation is indicated. Water is shown as black. Thailand Remote Sensing Centre, National Research Council of Thailand. Reproduced by permission

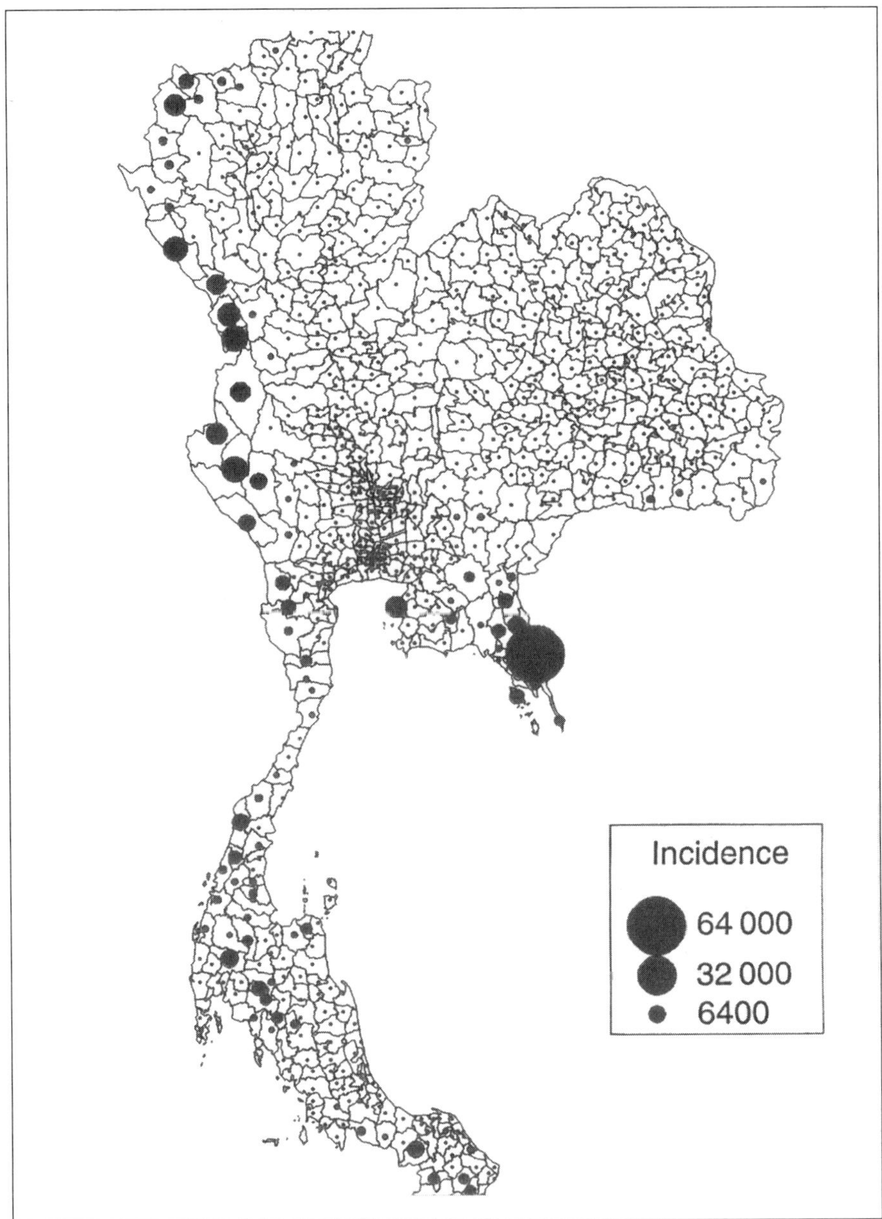

Figure 7.2 New malaria cases in Thailand in 1991

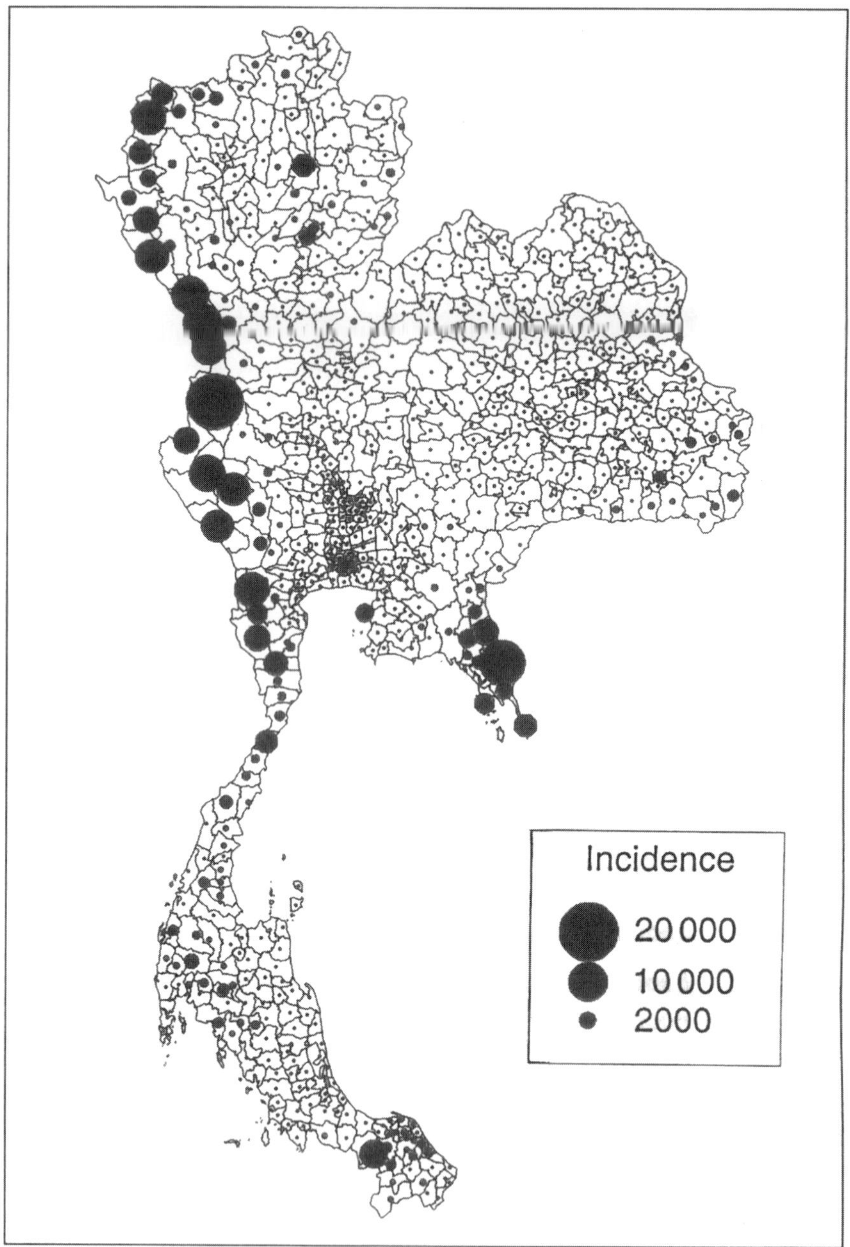

Figure 7.3 New malaria cases in Thailand in 1994

Table 7.1 Percentage land use by category in Chantaburi and Kanchanaburi Districts, Thailand: 1986–1995

Land use	1986	1989	1990	1991	1995
Chantaburi District					
Forest	37.0	30.4		34.1	23.5
Paddy	6.0	3.5		3.2	2.9
Rubber/orchard	18.5	31.9		25.2	25.2
Field crops	36.3	22.3		29.5	39.3
Other	2.0	11.9		8.0	9.1
Total	100	100		100	100
Kanchanaburi District					
Forest	59.6		62.2		
Paddy	3.9		9.9		
Sugarcane	14.2		15.5		
Other	22.2		12.3		
Total	100		100		

province bordering Myanmar (Burma), but a significant incidence in the east, on the border with Cambodia, can also be seen. It was possible to eliminate possible errors from presumptive classification of case origin (inherent in data from 1986–94) for 1995 by means of patient interview at selected malaria clinics in these provinces. For every person coming to the clinic with confirmed malaria during one calendar year 1996–97, efforts were made to establish where the infection had been contracted (through specific information on the movements of the person in the previous two weeks) and the residence of the patient. This information allowed an assessment to be made of the percentage of malaria cases that were likely to have been contracted in different ecotypes.

Table 7.1 summarizes changes in land use between 1986 and 1995. The total land area devoted to forest fell from 37% to 23.5% between 1986 and 1995 in Chantaburi District on the Thai–Cambodian border, and from 59.6% to 23.5% in Kanchanaburi District between 1986 and 1990 on the Thai–Myanmar border. Some of the land made available by deforestation was converted to commercial tree crops; rubber/orchards increased from 18.5% to 25.2% between 1986 and 1995 in Chantaburi District. (Land-use maps are still being evaluated in Kanchanaburi District.)

Table 7.2 provides information on man-biting rates over 10 months in different commercial tree crop plantations and results of searches for *An. dirus* larvae in various plantations. Man-biting rates indicate the potential for active transmission in new tree plantations—specifically in rubber plantations and orchards. The data on larval collections show that these plantations provide an effective breeding habitat for *An. dirus*. The malaria case data reflect the high percentage of cases associated with natural forest, orchards and rubber plantations.

Table 7.2 *An. dirus* collections and risk of malaria by habitat (10 months of collection 1995–96)

Habitat	Human biting rates: Number of *An. dirus* collected/human/night	Larval collections	Malaria cases
Chantaburi Province			
Natural forest	1.4	+	23.4
Orchard	2.1	+	28.5
Rubber	1.4	+	14.7
House in orchard	0.[illegible]	–	NA
Kanchanaburi Province			
Natural forest	1.9	+	59.3
Orchard	0.7	+	10.6
Teak	2.5	+	0.93
Village in teak plantation	0.3	–	NA

NA, not applicable

Discussion

The results of this study suggest that natural forest—the 'natural' habitat for *An. dirus*—is not an obligatory habitat for the vector. The data obtained provide direct evidence that the vector is at least as efficient at transmitting malaria in new commercial tree crop plantations as in its natural habitat. Thus malaria, which has been indigenous to large areas of natural forest but which had disappeared with the forest, has re-emerged in response to investments in plantations which permit mosquito breeding and survival, as well as providing a steady supply of hosts to infect. When *An. dirus* recolonizes this substantially restored habitat, malaria returns as an occupational disease. These new colonies of *An. dirus* act as a reservoir of intense, unchecked malaria transmission, from which the workers who come to work during harvest periods can carry the parasite to their homes across Thailand.

However, the data obtained also suggest that there are variations in malaria transmission between different tree plantations because of variations in the ecological conditions created by different tree crops. An important, unanswered question raised by these findings is why the ecosystems created by certain monoculture tree plantations enhance transmission of malaria. The soil, water, fertilizer, pesticides and spacing requirements of single species tree crop production vary according to species and scale of production. The situation becomes more complex when different tree species are combined for economic or ecological reasons and when humans from non-malaria-endemic areas come into these plantations to work on a permanent or temporary basis. The process of commercial and small-scale tree crop development varies in labour requirements, and therefore the potential for human–vector contact, through the process of planting, maintenance and harvesting. These factors determine transmission potential.

Since *An. dirus* is the most important vector in south-east Asia, information on its adaptability to new re-created habitats applies throughout the region. The data obtained from these studies provide an explanation for recent regional epidemics within rubber plantations and equally, and perhaps more importantly, allow prediction of epidemics in those areas where large tracts of land of virgin forest are now being logged and converted to plantations, in response to world prices for the commodity.

Rubber plantations are on the increase throughout the region—in Vietnam, Cambodia, Myanmar and Thailand. In Myanmar, large tracts of natural forest are being cut and replaced with rubber plantations and new settlements are being established in these areas. This is a similar situation to that seen in Vietnam, where people were relocated in 1978 from North Vietnam to South Vietnam as a permanent labour force in very large State plantations. Thirteen years after the initial stands were created, a significant proportion of the many deaths from malaria reported in Vietnam occurred where trees had grown to the age at which they provided the ideal conditions for intense breeding of *An. dirus*. Non-immunes were exposed to very high levels of transmission and all age groups were at risk of illness and death. These rubber plantations provide an important economic benefit to the country. Had it been possible to predict their impact on malaria in advance, it might have been possible to institute preventive measures and thereby reduce their negative health impact.

In Myanmar and Thailand, workers are contracted by the day to collect resin, plant or maintain plantations. Each day that they are ill, they lose pay, and bear the cost of treatment, transport and hospitalization. In Vietnam, the rubber plantations are largely organized, State-owned enterprises with a permanent workforce who live alongside the plantations with their families. In these plantations, it is not merely the adults who are at risk, but also children. Because the enterprise loses from each non-productive work day, the plantation workers and their families are provided with hospital care, treatment, diagnostic facilities and preventive measures by the rubber plantation.

Case 2. Ethiopia: microdams and afforestation

In 1994, a major rural development programme in Tigray, called 'Sustainable Agriculture and Environmental Rehabilitation in Tigray' (SEAERT), was initiated as an important way of changing the agrarian system of Tigray to one geared to widespread irrigation, in order to minimize dependence on rain-fed systems and to provide a means for self-sufficiency in food production. A component of the project was water resource development—the building of over

500 microdams, and the terracing of 200 000 hectares of agricultural and agro-forestry lands as part of the task of improving soil conservation and farm management practices. To date, 65 of the 500 microdams have been built, financed largely by local resources.

The construction of these microdams is expected to result in positive microclimatic and environmental changes. Change from rain-fed agriculture to small-scale irrigation through the use of run-off harvesting in microdams should increase agricultural productivity. Irrigation should permit the production of 4.5 tonnes more wheat and an additional 16 tonnes of potatoes per year per hectare of irrigated land. Achieving this potential would signify an increase in land productivity sufficient to feed an extra 930 000 people who are otherwise dependent upon food aid.

This agricultural development has been partially implemented in a malaria-endemic area. Malaria incidence within the area is normally seasonal, associated with the annual rains. Microdams are potentially an important breeding site for mosquitoes transmitting malaria, and the shade provided by afforestation could prolong the survival of such mosquitoes. Thus, implementing agencies and the Health Bureau in Tigray have been concerned that an unintended effect of this important rural agricultural development might be an increase in the incidence of malaria and a corresponding increase in illness and death among the resident population and among temporary and permanent migrants drawn into the project area for work.

The worst possible outcome would be a change in the epidemiological pattern of malaria from a seasonal to a perennial transmission cycle, increasing the incidence of malaria above the present level of one episode per year. An increased rate of illness and death among non-immune adults (the most productive group in economic terms) would reduce their productivity, particularly that of migrants drawn in from other areas. This, in turn, might lead to poor operation of the drainage of the irrigation systems, an increase in soil salinity and abandonment of irrigated lands. An investment which could have yielded a high positive rate of return to the economy might result in a loss, or a less than profitable yield.

Methodology

Because of the concerns expressed above, the World Health Organization's Special Programme for Research and Training in Tropical Diseases (TDR) designed a research project to detect whether construction of dams and afforestation increase transmission of malaria, and whether this increased transmission brings about a higher level of disease (clinical events). Developed by TDR, but funded largely by the Swedish SIDA, the project has involved the longitudinal monitoring of malaria incidence in the susceptible population through four paired, quarterly incidence surveys carried out in a population of

7400 children below the age of 10 years. Each pair of surveys has been implemented 30 days apart. The conversion of negative cases on day 1 to positive cases on day 30 gives an incidence rate per month. A history of fever was obtained and the temperature recorded at the time that each mass blood survey was done. Fever cases occurring between day 1 and day 30 were examined for malaria so as to obtain information on the incidence of symptomatic infection.

Results

Based on 6166 paired observations in children resident in villages near the dams–reafforestation, the incidence of malaria was calculated at 3.18%, compared to an incidence of 0.54% in children resident in villages away from the dams–reafforestation. This difference is highly significant ($z = 6.9$; $p < 0.0001$).

Discussion

In much of Africa, the epidemiology of malaria is dictated by climate and altitude. In the Sahel region and in dry land areas of Eastern Africa, malaria transmission is at its peak during the short rainy season. In these areas, harvesting of water for irrigation purposes in the dry season might result in a high density of anopheline mosquitoes and high transmission of malaria. Irrigation schemes which provide water during the dry season have the potential to increase malaria by providing suitable breeding sites for anopheline mosquitoes as well as extending risk exposure to a different, possibly larger, population employed in agricultural production as part of the irrigation scheme.

However, transmission potential is linked critically with ambient temperature and humidity. Research in The Gambia has shown that although vector densities increased with irrigation during the dry season, the incidence of malaria did not increase correspondingly (Lindsay *et al*, 1991). It was hypothesised that the risk of malaria did not increase despite sufficient vector densities either because of the reduced longevity of *An. gambiae* mosquitoes in the dry season or because of high temperatures which were lethal to parasite development. The daily survival rate of the mosquito is, all other things being equal, the one which causes the greatest rise in inoculation rates (Onori and Grab, 1980). Poor daily survival may reflect the extremely high temperatures and low ambient humidity experienced during the dry season, when temperatures can rise to 42°C in the shade and when mosquitoes might be exposed to temperatures over 35°C for several hours each day.

Unlike findings in the Sahel region, data from semi-arid areas of Ethiopia indicate that mosquito survival is greater in conditions where the relative humidity in small areas is increased because of the simultaneous afforestation accompanying microdam development. Trees provide shade, increase water retention in the soil, and inhibit evapotranspiration and temperature rises. Lower temperatures are more conducive to mosquito survival and therefore to transmission potential.

Conclusion

Infectious and parasitic diseases remain the major causes of death in much of the world. Malaria alone is associated with 300–3500 million clinical illnesses per year and one million deaths in children. When ecological changes cause a heightened risk for an infectious disease, the result can be illness and death in epidemic form. Epidemics are the most feared and costly expression of a disease for three reasons. First, the unexpected nature of the problem means that people will die because the cause of the epidemic is not appreciated immediately, and appropriate emergency resource allocation can be made only following confirmation of cause. Frequently, manpower and stocks of drugs and other supplies, allocated on the basis of historical data, are not sufficient and need to be augmented in the epidemic area. Secondly, epidemics place all age groups at risk of enhanced morbidity and mortality. Unlike situations of stable malaria (either seasonal or perennial) where immunity to infection is acquired over time as a result of a stable and predictable exposure to infection, in epidemic malaria a high intensity of infection places even those with some level of acquired immunity at greater risk of clinical illness and death. Thirdly, the costs to the health system are extremely high because of the speed with which decisions are required; speedy actions usually have a high financial cost.

It is very difficult for the health system to control an epidemic whose cause is outside its jurisdiction. It picks up the cost, with no ability to eliminate the source. In circumstances where ecological or environmental changes undertaken for compelling agricultural and economic reasons give the vector and parasite an advantage that is accentuated through the provision of regular human blood meals—as dictated by agricultural demands: planting, weeding, maintenance and harvest—epidemic malaria can be the result. The benefits of the investment will be obtained by the agricultural sector, while the costs are incurred by the health sector which has little or no ability to eliminate or mitigate the cause. This disequilibrium can be sustained as long as the latter cannot convince the former to internalize the costs, i.e. to reduce the benefits to the extent required to mitigate the negative health impact.

In the example given in Case 1, the costs of malaria are borne by the workers, and not internalized by the commercial tree crop plantations, as when temporary workers hired on a daily basis (during seasons when intensive work is required) fall ill with malaria, they are not paid and must, in addition, bear the costs of treatment and cure. Because the plantations do not bear this cost and lose little (except perhaps the search cost to obtain a replacement) they have no incentive to introduce or mitigate the levels of malaria incurred. In the example given in Case 2 above, the development investment yields a health benefit and cost. Improved food yields should increase nutrition and health; the increases in malaria constitute an adverse impact upon health which could be sufficiently large for the people to abandon their lands.

The investment in both examples is funded partially by national funds but international loans have been sought. For the lending agency, the investment decision requires a thorough appraisal of the project's benefits and costs, in financial and economic values, to facilitate calculation of the project's internal rate of return. Any predicted health impacts need to be quantified and, in order to estimate their effect on the project's economic viability, they have to be valued. Such valuation is complex, especially in those cases where the project affects mortality rather than morbidity, necessitating an estimation of the value of human life.

The data given in this paper provide two of the first examples of situations in which the epidemiological impact of investments in agricultural projects have been documented. This information is essential to project design and appraisal for two reasons. First, the data can be extrapolated to the region because of the regional nature of the vector. Secondly, quantitative epidemiological data are essential to place economic costs (values) on health risks. The relevant data in project appraisal are the incremental effects solely attributable to the development in question, assuming that these can be separated from the baseline situation; this depends upon a good research design and is not always an easy task. In extreme cases, the inclusion of these quantified health impacts could nullify the other economic benefits of a project; in other cases, the exercise would enable an informed judgement to be made of the size of mitigation programme that is justifiable.

Without an understanding of the epidemiological and economic costs and benefits of the investment, the health costs and the value of mitigating these costs cannot be put into perspective.

References

Lindsay SW, Wilkins HA, Zieler HA, Daly RJ, Petrarca V, Byass P. Ability of *Anopheles gambiae* mosquitoes to transmit malaria during the dry and wet seasons in an area of irrigated rice cultivation in The Gambia. *Journal of Tropical Medicine and Hygiene*, 1991; **94**: 313–324

Linthicum KJ, Thimasarn K, Nualchawee K *et al.* Effect of vegetation cover on the transmission of malaria in Thailand. Abstract no. 374, Annual Meeting of the American Society of Tropical Medicine and Hygiene. *American Journal of Tropical Medicine and Hygiene – Supplement*, 1996; **55**: 70.

Onori E, Grab B. Indicators for forecasting of malaria epidemics. *Bulletin of the World Health Organization*, 1980; **58**: 91–98

Rosenberg R, Andre RA, Somchit L. Highly efficient dry season transmission of malaria in Thailand. *Transactions of the Royal Society of Tropical Medicine and Hygiene*, 1990; **84**: 22–28

8
Ebola haemorrhagic fever: emerging or not?

Pierre E. Rollin, Thomas G. Ksiazek, Anthony Sanchez and Sherif R. Zaki*

*Special Pathogens Branch and *Infectious Disease Pathology Activity, National Center for Infectious Diseases, Centers for Disease Control and Prevention, Atlanta, GA, USA*

The filoviruses, Marburg and Ebola, are the aetiological agents of similar diseases that result in high mortality and frequent nosocomial transmission in hospital and laboratory settings. Marburg virus was the first described member of the family *Filoviridae*. The virus was isolated in 1967 during a severe outbreak of a syndrome that included fever and haemorrhage in Marburg and Frankfurt, Germany, and in Belgrade, former Yugoslavia. Thirty-three cases and seven deaths occurred among vaccine-production workers, medical personnel, and family members attending patients (Peters *et al*, 1996). These same transmission patterns were also observed in 1976 during two large outbreaks of Ebola haemorrhagic fever in Africa. These epidemiological features have remained characteristic for *Filoviridae* over the past 30 years. The Reston serotype of Ebola virus stands apart in its absence of lethality for humans.

The discovery of Ebola virus and epidemics of the infection

All outbreaks of Ebola haemorrhagic fever have been in tropical Africa or in the Philippines, although with some secondary cases or cases among imported primates in temperate zones (Table 8.1).

In July and September 1976, two massive haemorrhagic fever epidemics began in Nzara (southern Sudan) and Yambuku (northern Zaire), with estimated case-fatality ratios of 53% (estimated 284 cases) and 88% (estimated 318 cases), respectively. Two serologically and genetically distinct viruses were isolated from patients in these outbreaks and were named Ebola virus (after a small river in north-western Zaire).

New and Resurgent Infections: Prediction, Detection and Management of Tomorrow's Epidemics.
Edited by B. Greenwood and K. De Cock. Published 1998 John Wiley & Sons Ltd.

Table 8.1 Ebola haemorrhagic fever outbreaks, 1976–1996

Virus serotype	Location	Year	Month	Cases (case–fatality ratio)	Epidemiology
Ebola Zaire	Yambuku, Zaire	1976	September	318 (88%)	Unknown origin. Spread by close contact and by reutilization of materials in health care centres
Ebola Sudan	Nzara, Sudan	1976	August	284 (53%)	Unknown origin. Spread thought to be mainly by close contact. Nosocomial transmission and infection of medical care personnel
Ebola Sudan	England	1976	November	1 (0%)	Laboratory infection by needle-stick
Ebola Zaire	Tandala, Zaire	1977	June	1 (100%)	Single case in missionary hospital
Ebola Sudan	Nzara, Sudan	1979	July	34 (65%)	Recurrent outbreak at the same site as the 1976 epidemic
Ebola Reston	Reston, USA	1989–1990	November	4 (0%)	Introductions of virus into US quarantine facility with imported monkeys from the Philippines
Ebola Reston	Siena, Italy	1992	March	0 (0%)	Introduction with monkeys derived from same export facility in the Philippines as 1989
Ebola Côte d'Ivoire	Tai, Côte d'Ivoire	1994	November	1 (0%)	Identified retrospectively
Ebola Zaire	Mékouka, Gabon	1994	December	49 (59%)	Identified retrospectively
Ebola Zaire	Kikwit, Zaire	1995 1996	December January	317 (80%)	Unknown origin. Spread by close contact. Urban and hospital outbreak
Ebola Zaire	Mayibout, Gabon	1996	February	31 (67.7%)	First cases were in contact with an infected chimpanzee.
Ebola Zaire	Booué, Gabon	1996	July	61 (75%)	First case hunter, several familial generations
Ebola Zaire	South Africa	1996	October	2 (50%)	Identified retrospectively when the fatal second case occurred. First case was in contact with Ebola patients in Gabon
Ebola Reston	Manila, Philippines	1996	February ?	0 (0%)	Same export facility involved 1989 and 1992
Ebola Reston	Alice, USA	1996	March	0 (0%)	Introduction with monkeys derived from same export facility in the Philippines as 1989

The Sudan outbreak started among three employees of a cotton factory in Nzara and spread, initially at a low rate, from patients to close relatives by contamination during nursing care (WHO, 1978b). Some patients were hospitalized in the town of Maridi, where a subsequent hospital epidemic led to the dissemination of the virus throughout the town. No contact with a previous case could be established for 21% of the cases in Nzara, compared with the well documented links of transmission for all but five of of the 203 patients investigated in Maridi. The clinical manifestations of the disease were distinct and relatively easy to identify in the epidemic context.

The Zaire outbreak started at the beginning of September 1976 in the Yambuku Mission Hospital (YMH), which remained the major source of dissemination of the disease until it was closed at the end of September (WHO, 1978a). Secondary cases occurred among relatives and health care personnel. Major risk factors early in the epidemic included receipt of one or more injections at YMH and, later, close contact with a patient. Fifty-eight of about 250 villages in the epidemic area recorded cases, with fewer than five cases per village in 64% of the affected villages. The majority of these affected villages were located along roads running east and west of the mission. One patient was evacuated to Kinshasa and was the origin of secondary and tertiary cases. Only four of the 17 staff members at the YMH escaped infection. Virus transmission was interrupted by using disposable instruments and by isolation of patients in their villages. An intensive search for undetected cases in the north-eastern region of Zaire was unable to show a link between epidemics in the Maridi–Nzara (Sudan) and Yambuku (Zaire) areas. Further laboratory studies confirmed the serologic and genetic differences between the virus strains isolated during the two outbreaks. Search for a virus reservoir was inconclusive.

A severe case associated with laboratory infection by needle stick was reported in 1976 in England, and a single fatal case occurred in 1977 in Tandala (northern Zaire), not far to the west of the location of the original outbreak (Heymann *et al*, 1980). Epidemiological investigations revealed some possible previous clinical infections with Ebola virus in this area and a 7% seroprevalence among local residents, by using an immunofluorescent antibody (IFA) test of uncertain sensitivity and specificity.

In 1979, another outbreak occurred at Nzara in which 34 cases (22 deaths) of Ebola haemorrhagic fever were confirmed (Baron *et al*, 1983). The index patient had been employed in the Nzara textile factory where the 1976 outbreak originated. During his hospitalization, in early August, this patient became the focal point of dissemination of infection to nurses, other patients, and patients' families. Providing nursing care and having direct physical contact with patients were responsible for most of the secondary cases. The outbreak was brought under control when barrier nursing practices were implemented. No further evidence of Ebola virus disease in Africa was seen until 17 years later.

The IFA method, developed during the previous epidemics, was used to conduct serosurveys among different populations in several central African countries, and in ecoclimatic zones (Meunier *et al*, 1987a; 1987b; Gonzalez *et al*, 1989). Significant variation in the seroprevalence was observed, ranging between 0 and 20%. These results, obtained in the absence of typical epidemic disease, led to different hypotheses to account for this pattern of seroreactivity: (1) the presence of non-pathogenic Ebola strains with a wide range of clinical manifestations, (2) cross-reactivity with another filovirus; or (3) poor specificity of the IFA assay.

During the autumn of 1989, several cynomolgus macaques (*Macaca fascicularis*) that had recently been imported into a US primate quarantine facility from a commercial farm in the Philippines died from an illness suggestive of viral haemorrhagic fever; infection with simian haemorrhagic fever (SHF) virus was suspected as the cause (Dalgard *et al*, 1992). Unexpectedly, in addition to SHF virus, a new serotype of Ebola virus, called Ebola Reston virus, was isolated. Epidemiological investigations traced the origin of this outbreak to a single facility of an exporter of non-human primates. The same source was responsible for the subsequent exportation of Ebola virus-infected monkeys to the USA in 1990, to Siena, Italy, in 1992, and once again to the USA in 1996. The origin of the contamination of this exporter's facility remains unknown. Several valuable diagnostic tests were developed during and after these outbreaks.

In November 1994, a primate ethologist was infected with a new serotype of Ebola virus while performing a necropsy on a chimpanzee found dead in a national park in western Côte d'Ivoire (LeGuenno *et al*, 1995). In the preceding weeks, an unusually high mortality among the chimpanzees in the national park had been recorded. The high mortality and rapid course of the disease argue strongly against a reservoir role for these primates. Further ecological studies are planned to investigate the relationship between chimpanzees and their environment. In May 1995, a massive epidemic affected the residents in and around Kikwit, in the south-central part of Zaire (Muyembe *et al*, 1995). The epidemic started in the town in January but remained unnoticed until late April, when it spread rapidly as a result of nosocomial spread in the local general hospital. The epidemic resulted in approximately 300 cases, with an 80% mortality (Khan *et al*, 1996). The use of the enzyme-linked immunosorbent assay (ELISA) antigen and IgM detection tests developed at the US Army Medical Research Institute for Infectious Diseases (USAMRIID) laboratories allowed rapid confirmation of suspected Ebola haemorrhagic fever cases by the Special Pathogens laboratories at the Centers for Disease Control and Prevention (CDC). An international response helped to control the epidemic. The clinical manifestations and the pattern of interhuman transmission observed in the previous epidemics were confirmed and extended during investigation of the 1995 outbreak. Testing of serial specimens collected in parallel with clinical observations provided a timely and accurate measure of infection and confirmed the reliability of the ELISA. The finding of Ebola antigens in human skin specimens by immunohistochemistry

(Zaki *et al*, unpublished data) provided the basis for a new and practical surveillance test for Ebola haemorrhagic fever. An ecological investigation conducted from June to August 1995 produced an extensive collection of mammals, birds and arthropods. The delay between the infection of the suspected index patient in January and the start of the ecological studies did not diminish expectations that a putative reservoir carrying the virus and/or having detectable antibody might be found. The processing of the thousands of specimens collected is still under way, but so far without any positive results for Ebola virus.

In nearby Gabon, three separate outbreaks occurred in late 1994, and in February and July 1996 respectively, each caused by slightly different strains of the Zaire subtype of Ebola virus. The first and the second episodes started during the rainy season, December and February, while the third began during the dry season (July) (Amblard *et al*, 1997; Georges-Courbot *et al*, 1997b; WHO, 1978a; 1996a; 1996b; 1997a; 1997b). As in Côte d'Ivoire, deaths of non-human primates were reported during these three outbreaks in Gabon. Dead chimpanzees and gorillas had been found in the local forest during the autumn of 1994. All the primary infections among humans in the spring 1996 outbreak were associated with butchering and cooking a dead chimpanzee. For the third outbreak, the index patient was a hunter, living in a forest camp in the Booué area not far from a place where an Ebola-virus-positive, dead chimpanzee had been found.

Molecular biology of filoviruses

Marburg and Ebola viruses, the only members of the family *Filoviridae*, are composed of a helical nucleocapsid covered by an envelope with glycoprotein spikes protruding from the virion surface. In electron microscopy preparations, both Ebola and Marburg viruses appear as long, filamentous, and sometimes branched forms. The length of virions varies greatly, but the diameter is uniform (80 nm). The virion contains one molecule of non-infectious, linear, negative-sense, single-stranded RNA coding for seven structural proteins. Four of them (the nucleoprotein, VP30, VP35 and the polymerase) are associated with the RNA to form a ribonucleocapsid complex. The three remaining structural proteins are membrane-associated: the glycoprotein, VP24 and VP40 (Feldmann *et al*, 1993). The glycoprotein gene has been used to define the relationship of Ebola viruses to one another and to Marburg viruses. While no subtypes have been detected in Marburg virus, four subtypes of Ebola virus have been identified (Zaire, Sudan, Reston, Ivory Coast) (Figure 8.1). Phylogenetic analysis clearly differentiates the Marburg from the Ebola lineages, and each of the Ebola subtypes represents a monophyletic lineage. The Ebola Zaire subtype has remained very similar over the 20-year span of the outbreaks, and the large distance between Yambuku, Kikwit, and the northern part of Gabon suggests a closely related (if not identical) reservoir (Sanchez *et al*, 1996).

A feature of the glycoprotein gene that may be important to the survival of

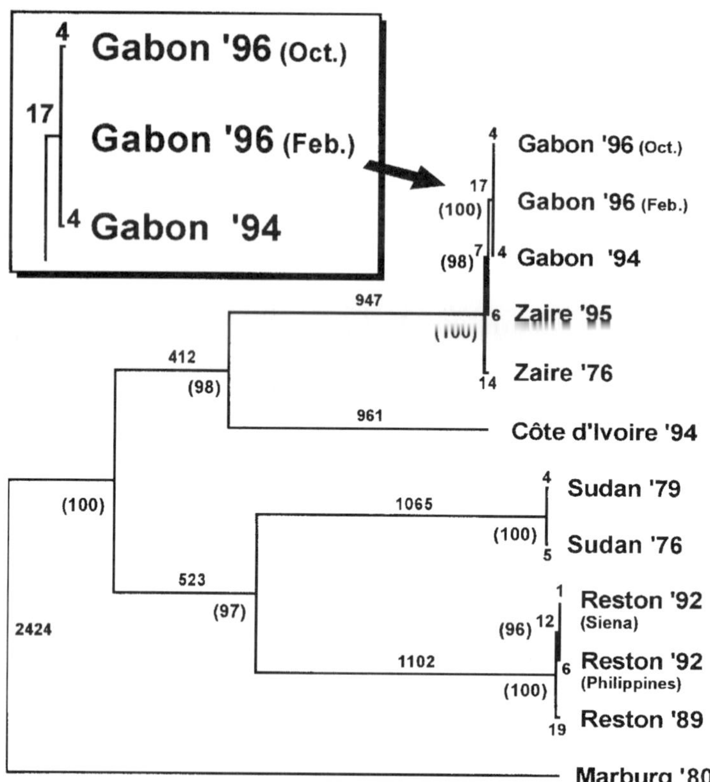

Figure 8.1 Phylogenetic tree showing the relationship between the Ebola viruses that caused outbreaks of disease in Gabon and previously described filoviruses. The entire coding region for the glycoprotein gene of the viruses shown was used in maximum parsimony analysis, and a single most parsimonious tree was obtained. Numbers in parentheses indicate bootstrap confidence values for branch points and were generated from 500 replicates (heuristic search). Branch length values are also shown. Source: Georges-Courbot *et al*, 1997a

Ebola viruses in the natural host is the organisation of the coding region. A small non-structural glycoprotein is the primary gene product, while the larger structural glycoprotein is expressed through transcriptional editing (encoded in two frames). The small glycoprotein is secreted and may interact with the host's cellular immune system and might also play a role in the pathogenesis of human infections (Sanchez *et al*, 1996).

Clinical manifestations and treatment

Symptoms and signs

After an incubation of between four and 10 days, Ebola haemorrhagic fever, like Marburg disease, starts with an abrupt onset of fever, severe frontal headache, malaise, and myalgia or back pain. Deterioration over the following two to three days is heralded by pharyngitis and sore throat, severe nausea, vomiting, and profuse diarrhoea and prostration. A cutaneous rash is obvious on white skin but can be difficult to identify on dark-skinned patients. Typical late signs associated with a poor prognosis are tachypnoea and bleeding, including epistaxis, haematemeses, melaena, petechiae, ecchymoses, uncontrolled bleeding from venepuncture sites, hiccups, oliguria and shock. Death usually occurs six to nine days after the onset of clinical disease. Convalescence is slow, often taking five weeks or more, and is marked by weight loss and prostration. It is sometimes associated with arthritis, conjunctivitis, hearing loss, or orchitis. Clinical laboratory findings based on non-human primate experiments and a few human reports include an early lymphopaenia, subsequent neutrophilia and a marked thrombocytopenia accompanied by abnormal platelet aggregation. Serum enzyme levels are elevated, typically with AST exceeding ALT, and with alkaline phosphatase and bilirubin levels normal or only moderately elevated (Peters *et al*, 1996).

Differential diagnosis

Outside the course of a known epidemic, in which clinical suspicion is sustained by the epidemiological context, other possible diagnoses of non-specific febrile illness are difficult to eliminate clinically. Treatable infectious diseases should be excluded or covered by specific therapy. Among the wide range of parasitic, bacterial, rickettsial and viral diseases to be considered, those that should first come to mind are malaria, typhoid fever and shigellosis. The occurrence of clusters of cases with evidence of person-to-person transmission among close contacts and hospital staff should be sufficient grounds for making a presumptive diagnosis of a viral haemorrhagic fever (due to Ebola, Marburg, Lassa or Crimean–Congo viruses) and for instituting strict barrier-nursing procedures.

Treatment

No specific treatment is available for Marburg and Ebola haemorrhagic fevers. Ribavirin, an antiviral drug used to treat several other haemorrhagic fevers, has no *in vitro* effect on Marburg and Ebola viruses and is unlikely to be of any clinical value. Human convalescent-phase plasma has been proposed and used in Zaire and, in spite of lack of any clinical or experimental data regarding its efficacy, its use would be reasonable provided it was available and free of known blood-borne pathogens. Hyperimmune horse serum has also been used in a non-human primate model with contradicting results on protection (Mikhailov *et al*, 1994; Jahrling *et al*, 1996). Intensive supportive care is most important; prevention of shock, cerebral oedema, renal failure, platelet and clotting factor depletion, bacterial superinfection, hypoxia and hypotension may be life-saving. Care is complicated by the need for isolation and protection of medical and nursing personnel. Recommendations require the wearing of personal protective clothing (including gloves, gown and mask), adherence to strict barrier-nursing techniques, and use of aerosol personal protection when feasible (Centers for Disease Control and Prevention, 1995).

Diagnosing filovirus diseases

Filovirus disease should be included in the differential diagnostic of acute, febrile illness in anyone who has recently travelled in rural sub-Saharan Africa, particularly when haemorrhagic manifestations are present. The differential diagnosis includes arboviral infections, including yellow fever, chikungunya fever, Rift Valley fever and Crimean–Congo haemorrhagic fever, and other viral illnesses such as Lassa fever and fulminant viral hepatitis. Aetiological diagnosis is nearly impossible for the physician presented with a single case of haemorrhagic fever in rural Africa without laboratory support. However, when a cluster of cases occurs with a prodromal febrile illness with or without a high proportion of haemorrhagic cases, and when transmission from person to person is observed among close contacts and hospital staff, a presumptive diagnosis of viral haemorrhagic fever must be made, and containment procedures must be put in place. Diagnostic specimens should be handled with extreme caution and sent to an appropriate laboratory, keeping in mind that the infectivity of a virus suspension is stable at room temperature, especially if the solution contains proteins, as found in serum or blood, but that virus is inactivated by heat, lipid solvents, gamma-irradiation, betapropiolactone, hypochlorite, and phenolic disinfectants.

Direct detection of virus or its constituents can be achieved using several different techniques. Immunofluorescence applied to impression smears of tissues, antigen-detection ELISA, immunohistochemistry, and the polymerase chain reaction (PCR) have all been used to demonstrate filovirus material in clinical materials. Ebola viruses are not difficult to isolate and propagate in cell culture, provided that a sensitive cell line is used but, on primary isolation, the viruses are not extremely cytopathic (Peters *et al*, 1996). The best way to confirm their isolation is either to stain the culture with a specific antibody, or to check the cells by electron microscopy for the characteristic morphologic features of filovirus virions and nucleocapsids. The growth of the virus should be contemplated only in a high-containment laboratory. A skin biopsy kit was developed and used as a surveillance and post-mortem confirmation tool in Zaire and Gabon (Lloyd *et al*, 1996). The principle is based on the recent finding that in fatal cases, Ebola virus antigen is present in large quantities in the dermal endothelial cells and connective tissue.

Until recently, the serologic diagnosis of filovirus disease was made by the IFA, both for serosurveys and diagnosis of acute suspected cases. However, this technique has some problems with specificity and sensitivity. Most patients who die of Ebola haemorrhagic fever have a very high titre of circulating virus and antigens but no antibody, resulting in a false negative diagnostic result for Ebola virus if IFA is used solely for diagnosis. An IgM capture assay can be used to diagnose acute infections with Ebola and Marburg viruses in non-human primates and in humans correctly. A direct IgG ELISA should replace the IFA for seroprevalence studies.

Pathology and pathogenesis

A number of experimental primate studies and a few human necropsy tissues collected mainly during the 1995 outbreak in Zaire have shown that several mechanisms could be responsible for the pathophysiological changes observed during Marburg and Ebola virus infections. Gross pathological changes in fatal Marburg and Ebola haemorrhagic fever cases include haemorrhage into skin, mucous membranes, visceral organs, and the lumen of the stomach and intestines. Microscopic changes in Marburg and Ebola virus cases include focal necrosis of liver, lymphoid organs, kidneys, testes and ovaries. Most prominent is focal necrosis of the liver parenchyma. Involved hepatocytes often contain large eosinophilic intracytoplasmic inclusion bodies, which are coincident with masses of viral nucleocapsids observed by electron microscopy. Within necrotic foci, there are Councilman-like bodies but very few inflammatory cells. Immunohistochemical study has shown large deposits of viral antigens in hepatocytes and Kuppfer cells and free in the intercellular connective tissues. Endothelial cells are heavily infected in the liver as well as in other tissues (Zaki *et al*, 1996).

Filoviruses can directly infect cultured endothelial cells as well as macrophages, producing a cytopathic effect. Supernatants from Marburg virus-infected macrophages contain TNF-alpha and can increase the permeability of uninfected endothelial cells in the presence of minimal quantities of oxygen-free radicals. TNF-alpha can result in secondary activation of secretion of other important mediators (Feldmann *et al*, 1996).

Transmission

Transmission from patient to patient within hospital settings has been associated with reuse of unsterilized needles and syringes (WHO, 1978a). High rates of secondary transmission have also occurred among health-care workers and among family members of patients who provided nursing care without appropriate barrier precautions to prevent exposure to virus-containing blood or other body fluids. The specific risk associated with contact with various body fluids has not been defined because most care-givers who acquired infection had multiple contacts with various body fluids. A study of transmission among household members of infected persons was done in Kikwit (Dowell *et al*, unpublished data). The risk of developing Ebola haemorrhagic fever was highest among spouses of the primary household case and among family members older than 18 years. Of the 28 secondary cases, 12 had direct contact with blood, vomitus, or stool of the ill person during hospitalization, and 17 shared the same hospital bed. Of 78 household members who had no direct physical contact with the primary household case during the period of clinical illness, none developed Ebola haemorrhagic fever.

Available data suggest that the risk for infection is highest among persons who have direct contact with a patient in the later stages of illness, characterized by vomiting, diarrhoea, shock, and occasionally haemorrhage. Transmission also occurs frequently during ritual manipulation of corpses. No cases of Ebola haemorrhagic fever have been reported from persons whose contact with an infected patient occurred only during the incubation period (before the patient developed fever).

Although aerosol transmission has not been implicated in human outbreaks to date, it cannot be discounted because filoviruses can be transmitted to non-human primates by experimental or accidental aerosol exposure (Jaax *et al*, 1995). Furthermore, the disease caused by the Reston subtype of Ebola virus among quarantined monkeys during the 1989–90 outbreak was transmitted by droplets and perhaps small-particle aerosols (Dalgard *et al*, 1992; Peters *et al*, 1994). Marburg and Ebola virions have also been identified in alveoli of experimentally infected monkeys and human lung specimens obtained during the Kikwit episode (Zaki, unpublished data).

Epidemiology and natural reservoir

The origin and the natural history of Marburg and Ebola viruses remain a mystery. It seems likely that they can be transmitted to humans from an animal or arthropod reservoir (Peters *et al*, 1994). The question of whether non-human primates might be the primary reservoir has been raised several times: during the original Marburg outbreak, then during the 1989–1990 outbreak of Reston virus from the Philippines, and more recently in Côte d'Ivoire and Gabon. This hypothesis was based on large serosurveys of non-human primates in which antibodies were detected by using an IFA test, but none of these results was confirmed when a more specific ELISA was used. Furthermore, the high lethality of filoviruses for non-human primates seems to indicate that, like humans, the animals constitute incidental victims of infection and are not true reservoir hosts.

The low density of non-human primates remaining in the wild would not be able to sustain the same kind of ongoing transmission of Ebola Reston virus observed for several months in a quasi-experimental situation in a Philippines primates breeding farm which maintained a high density of animals.

In some instances of Marburg virus infection, it was established that people who subsequently presented as primary cases had visited buildings or caves where numerous bats roosted, and it is known that one patient was bitten or stung by a presumed arthropod prior to developing Marburg disease. Even suggestions that filoviruses may be plant viruses have been made.

The fact that outbreaks of filovirus infections have been rare and have occurred in remote and widely dispersed geographic locations has complicated the search for the source of the viruses in nature. In addition, few laboratories can support the burden of field investigations for these infections. Following the recognition of the 1995 epidemic of Ebola fever in Kikwit, Zaire, teams of scientists, coordinated by the CDC in Atlanta, collected large numbers of vertebrate and arthropod specimens during June, July and August 1995. Another collection was made by a team from the National Institute for Virology in South Africa in January 1996. Approximately 3200 vertebrates, mostly mammals (e.g. *rodentia, chiroptera, insectivora*), and more than 30 000 invertebrates (e.g. mosquitoes, ticks) were collected, identified, sampled, and preserved in nitrogen in the field. The tissues were sent to CDC and USAMRIID for serological testing and virus isolation attempts in biosafety level 4 containment facilities. Because of the huge workload and the lack of some specific immune reagents for uncommon species, several hundred specimens remain to be processed. No antibody or virus isolates of filovirus have been obtained from the specimens tested, though several arenaviruses have been isolated from rodent tissues.

At the National Institute of Virology in South Africa, another approach to finding the reservoir was tried by performing pathogenicity studies with Ebola virus in representatives of different vertebrates, invertebrates and plants (Swanepoel *et al*, 1996). Thirty-three varieties of 24 species of plants and 19 species of vertebrates and invertebrates were experimentally inoculated with Ebola Zaire virus. Only fruit and insectivorous bats were found to support replication and circulation of high titres of virus; they did not show any clinical signs. Although nothing conclusive can be derived from this preliminary study, continued use of this approach can serve to focus studies on groups of animals capable of supporting replication of the virus. It is notable that the two species of Tadarid bats studied, and many other bats, have a distribution which overlaps the sites of known filovirus outbreaks in Africa, and the migratory habits of some species would facilitate dissemination of virus.

Is Ebola haemorrhagic fever an emerging viral disease?

Most of the 'new' viruses discovered have probably existed for centuries, escaping detection because they are found only in remote areas where, if humans do encounter them, disease goes undiagnosed because of poor or non-existent medical or diagnostic infrastructures. *Filoviridae* were recognised when Marburg virus was transported to Europe and when Ebola virus decimated the European medical staff of Yambuku Mission Hospital and more recently the staff of Kikwit General Hospital. Such a rapid, fatal disease with evident human-to-human transmission was the sentinel event for the recognition of Lassa fever in Nigeria in 1969. Lassa fever had never been observed or reported before in hospitals or medical centres in that country. It is also clear that, under some circumstances, a rampant epidemic of Ebola haemorrhagic fever can remain unrecognised and unreported to central authorities, as happened for several weeks in Nzara in 1976 or for several months in Kikwit, a town of several hundred thousand inhabitants, in 1995. Even when the viruses were introduced in the hospital setting, it took several generations of transmission and a dramatic loss of valuable medical personnel before the emergence was recognized and assistance was requested.

Several lines of evidence argue against recent genetic changes in the viruses converting them to a virulent form. Despite the fact that RNA viruses possess the potential for rapid evolution because of their high RNA polymerase error rate, Ebola virus seems to be particularly stable. Sequence analysis of the 1976 and 1995 strains of Ebola viruses from Zaire showed few modifications (less than 1.6% difference for the entire glycoprotein gene) (Sanchez *et al*, 1996). Recent analysis of viruses sequentially isolated during the Kikwit or the Gabon epidemics has shown that only one virus of unvarying sequence circulated during a given outbreak (Georges-Courbot *et al*, 1997a). The difference in the glycoprotein gene nucleotide sequence between the viruses of each epidemic was no more than four nucleotides. Viral virulence also seems to remain comparable because the reported case-mortality rates for outbreaks did not change appreciably between 1976 and 1996, varying between 55% and 88%. The consequences of the high mortality and the low incidence of the filovirus diseases, attested by an antibody prevalence equal to or close to zero in population studies, are that all populations must be considered naive. Thus, if the virus is reintroduced, they will be greatly at risk.

Environmental and behavioural factors can produce new circumstances in which filoviruses may flourish if they are introduced; these include urbanization, national conflicts leading to huge refugee populations, lack of resources (reuse of needles and syringes was clearly a factor for amplification in the Yambuku outbreak), and an inability to implement and sustain good barrier-nursing procedures in the medical centres, as occurred in the Kikwit episode. Good isolation procedures were the most important factor in avoiding nosocomial outbreaks following admission of a patient to hospital in Kinshasa during the

Zaire 1995 episode and following a recent case of Ebola in Johannesburg. Such procedures also contributed to the rapid control of hospital outbreaks in Kikwit in 1995, and in Makoukou, Gabon in the spring of 1996. Without knowledge of the natural reservoir of filoviruses, it is difficult to know whether agricultural changes or deforestation have had an effect on the emergence of the disease, but it is clear that these viruses are maintained in tropical sylvatic habitats, and human incursions and perturbations of these habitats will increase the probability of significant encounters with filoviruses.

The opportunities for disease emergence are also enhanced by the development of rapid travel. The mobility of both humans and sources of infection has increased tremendously in recent years. Without warning, infected patients or travellers with incubating disease can arrive in unexpected and unprepared places, as was demonstrated recently by the death of a nurse in Johannesburg, South Africa from Ebola. Ebola Reston-infected primates were imported to Reston in Virginia, Siena in Italy and Alice in Texas; only the existing quarantine regulations allowed early recognition and prevented the dissemination of these primates to further research or pharmaceutical laboratories.

Is the increased recognition of cases responsible for apparent emergence? The development of improved diagnostic tools and the better understanding of the patient immune response to Ebola virus infection certainly contribute to the perception of emergence. The rapid antigen and IgM detection ELISA and the molecular-based PCR can provide rapid results to a clinician suspecting an acute filovirus infection, compared with the several days required for virus isolation. Although rapid, the IFA test will not correctly identify most acute fatal cases. The skin biopsy test based on immunohistochemical detection of the virus can easily be used as a passive detection system of otherwise undiagnosed fatal Ebola haemorrhagic fever. The availability and the distribution of these tests and the limited number of experienced laboratories remain a problem.

Another factor in the 'emergent' awareness of Ebola disease is media coverage and the effect of such attention. In 1976, Yambuku was a nearly impossible location to reach, and satellite telephones had not yet been invented. As a result, the outbreak received no on-site media coverage. In 1995, the international press was at Kikwit airport to welcome the medical teams and to film the unloading of supplies.

What is the potential of filoviruses as emerging pathogens? These viruses have a number of undesirable characteristics: high primate pathogenicity, high host-to-host transmissibility, potential aerosol infectivity, lack of effective therapeutics, and research limited by safety requirements. On the other hand, their occurrence in geographically remote areas limits the risks to human populations. Realistic predictions on the emergence of filoviruses and strategies to protect the public are hindered by our limited knowledge of genetics, pathogenesis, natural history and reservoir of the filoviruses.

Acknowledgments

The authors thank John O'Connor for editorial assistance.

References

Amblard J, Obiang P, Edzang S, Prehaud C, Bouloy M, LeGuenno B. Identification of the Ebola virus in Gabon in 1994. *Lancet*, 1997; **349**: 181–182

Baron RC, McCormick JB, Zubeir OA. Ebola virus disease in southern Sudan: hospital dissemination and intra familial spread. *Bulletin of the World Health Organization*, 1983; **61**: 997–1003

Centers for Disease Control and Prevention. Update: Management of patients with suspected viral haemorrhagic fever—United States. *Morbidity and Mortality Weekly Report*, 1995; **44**: 475–479

Dalgard DW, Hardy RJ, Pearson SL *et al.* Combined simian haemorrhagic fever and Ebola virus infection in cynomolgus monkeys. *Laboratory Animal Science*, 1992; **42**: 152–157

Feldmann H, Klenk HD, Sanchez A. Molecular biology and evolution of filoviruses. *Archives of Virology*, 1993; **Suppl 7**: 81–100

Feldmann H, Bugany H, Mahner F, Klenk HD, Drenckhahn D, Schnittler HJ. Filovirus-induced endothelial leakage triggered by infected monocytes/macrophages. *Journal of Virology*, 1996; **70**: 2208–2214

Georges-Courbot MC, Sanchez A, Lu CY *et al.* Isolation and phylogenetic characterization of Ebola viruses causing different outbreaks in Gabon. *Emerging Infectious Diseases*, 1997a; **3**: 59–62

Georges-Courbot MC, Lu CY, Lansoud-Soukate J, Leroy E, Baize S. Isolation and partial molecular characterisation of a strain of Ebola virus during a recent epidemic of viral haemorrhagic fever in Gabon. *Lancet*, 1997b; **349**: 181

Gonzalez JP, Josse R, Johnson ED *et al.* Antibody prevalence against haemorrhagic fever viruses in randomized representative Central African populations. *Research in Virology*, 1989; **140**: 319–331

Heymann DL, Weisfeld JS, Webb PA, Johnson KM, Cairns T, Berquist H. Ebola haemorrhagic fever: Tandala, Zaire, 1977–1978. *Journal of Infectious Diseases*, 1980; **142**: 372–376

Jaax N, Jahrling P, Geisbert T *et al.* Transmission of Ebola virus (Zaire strain) to uninfected control monkeys in a biocontainment laboratory. *Lancet*, 1995; **346**: 1669–1671

Jahrling PB, Geisbert J, Swearengen JR *et al.* Passive immunization of Ebola virus-infected cynomolgus monkeys with immunoglobulin from hyperimmune horses. *Archives of Virology*, 1996; **11(Suppl)**: 135–140

Khan AS, Kipassa M, International Scientific and Technical Committee. Epidemiological features of the recent Ebola virus outbreaks: epidemiologic and control issues. Abstracts in: *International Colloquium on Ebola Virus Research, Antwerp, Belgium, Sept 4–7, 1996*

LeGuenno B, Formentry P, Wyers M, Gounon P, Walker F, Boesch C. Isolation and partial characterisation of a new strain of Ebola virus. *Lancet*, 1995; **345**: 1271–1274

Lloyd ES, Rollin PE, Zaki SR. Long term surveillance for Ebola in Africa. Abstracts in: *International Colloquium on Ebola Virus Research, Antwerp, Belgium, Sept 4–7, 1996*

Meunier DM, Dupont A, Madelon MC, Gonzalez JP, Ivanoff B. Serological study of haemorrhagic fevers in the province of Haut-Ogooue, Gabon. *Annales de l'Institut Pasteur/Virologie*, 1987a; **138**: 229–235

Meunier DM, Johnson ED, Gonzalez JP, Georges-Courbot MC, Madelon MC, Georges

AJ. Current serologic data on viral haemorrhagic fevers in the Central African Republic. *Bulletin de la Societé de Pathologie Exotique*, 1987b; **80**: 51–61
Mikhailov VV, Borisevich IV, Chernikova NK, Potryvaeva NV, Krasnianskii VP. The evaluation in hamadryas baboons of the possibility for the specific prevention of Ebola fever. *Voprosy Virusologii* (*Moskva*), 1994; **39**: 82–84
Muyembe T, Kipasa M. International Scientific and Technical Committee and WHO Collaborating Centre for Haemorrhagic Fevers. Ebola haemorrhagic fever in Kikwit, Zaire. *Lancet*, 1995; **345**: 1448
Peters CJ, Sanchez A, Feldmann H, Rollin PE, Nichol S, Ksiazek TG. Filoviruses as emerging pathogens. *Seminars in Virology*, 1994; **5**: 147–154
Peters CJ, Sanchez A, Rollin PE, Ksiazek TG, Murphy FA. Filoviridae: Marburg and Ebola viruses. In: Fields BN, Knipe DM, Howley PM (eds), *Fundamental Virology. 3rd edn.* Philadelphia, PA: Lippencott-Raven Publishers, 1996, pp 1161–1176
Sanchez A, Trappier SG, Mahy BWJ, Peters CJ, Nichol ST. The virion glycoproteins of Ebola viruses are encoded in two reading frames and are expressed through transcriptional editing. *Proceedings of the National Academy of Sciences of the USA*, 1996; **93**: 3602–3607
Swanepoel R, Leman PA, Burt FJ *et al.* Experimental inoculation of plants and animals with Ebola virus. *Emerging Infectious Diseases*, 1996; **2**: 321–325
World Health Organization (WHO). Ebola haemorrhagic fever in Zaire, 1976. *Bulletin of the World Health Organization*, 1978a; **56**: 271–293
World Health Organization (WHO). Ebola haemorrhagic fever in Sudan, 1976. Report of a WHO/International Study Team. *Bulletin of the World Health Organization*, 1978b; **56**: 247–270
World Health Organization (WHO). Ebola haemorrhagic fever—South Africa. *Weekly Epidemiological Record*, 1996a; **71**: 359
World Health Organization (WHO). Ebola haemorrhagic fever—Gabon. *Weekly Epidemiological Record*, 1996b; **71**: 366
World Health Organization (WHO). Ebola haemorrhagic fever—A summary of the outbreak in Gabon. *Weekly Epidemiological Record*, 1997a; **72**: 7–8
World Health Organization (WHO). Ebola haemorrhagic fever—Gabon. *Weekly Epidemiological Record*, 1997b; **72**: 23–24
Zaki SR, Greer PW, Goldsmith CS *et al.* Ebola virus haemorrhagic fever: pathologic, immunopathologic and ultrastructural study. Abstracts in: *International Colloquium on Ebola Virus Research. Antwerp, Belgium, Sept* 4–7, 1996

9
Population growth, urbanization, automobiles and aeroplanes: the dengue connection

Duane J. Gubler

Division of Vector-Borne Infectious Diseases, National Center for Infectious Diseases, Fort Collins, USA

In the past 50 years the world has experienced unprecedented population growth that continues unabated in the waning years of the 20th century. It is projected that by the year 2025, the global population will be 8.3 billion people, and by 2050, 10 billion people (Plant, 1996). Most of the recent population increase has occurred in urban centres of developing countries, which has resulted in uncontrolled and unplanned urbanization, especially in the tropics. Projections indicate that this trend will continue, with 95% of population growth in the next 25–30 years occurring in developing countries (World Resources Institute, 1996). Moreoever, it is estimated that by the year 2000, 39% of the global population will live in urban areas and that this will increase to 56% by the year 2025 (Knudsen and Sloof, 1992).

Coincident with these demographic changes have been societal changes that have had a marked influence on the movement of commerce and people. The car has greatly increased the mobility of humans and commodities on a local and regional basis, and the jet aeroplane has done the same for intercontinental movement of goods and people. While these changes reflect economic progress and have increased the standard of living in some respects, they have also had some disastrous effects on public health, especially in tropical developing countries of the world. The global resurgence of epidemic dengue fever and the emergence of dengue haemorrhagic fever are directly related to these changes. This chapter will review the changing epidemiology of dengue, some of the factors

New and Resurgent Infections: Prediction, Detection and Management of Tomorrow's Epidemics.
Edited by B. Greenwood and K. De Cock. Published 1998 John Wiley & Sons Ltd.

thought to be responsible for the dramatic increase in disease incidence and the prospects for reversing the trend of emergent disease in the future.

Natural history

Dengue fever (DEN) and dengue haemorrhagic fever (DHF) are caused by infection with dengue viruses. There are four closely related virus serotypes, DEN-1, DEN-2, DEN-3 and DEN-4; while these serotypes show extensive cross-reactivity in serological tests, they do not provide cross-protective immunity (Gubler, 1988). Thus, persons living in a DEN-endemic area can be infected with each of the four dengue serotypes during their lifetime.

Infection with dengue viruses is transmitted through the bite of infective female *Aedes spp* mosquitoes (Gubler, 1988). *Aedes aegypti*, the principal urban vector, is a small black-and-white, highly domesticated mosquito that prefers to lay its eggs in artificial water containers commonly found in urban areas of the tropics. Containers found in and around the home—such as those used for water storage, flower vases, old car tyres, buckets and various plastic containers—and other discarded objects that collect rainwater are examples. The adult mosquitoes are highly adapted to living with humans and are rarely noticed, preferring to rest indoors and to feed on humans during daylight hours in an unobtrusive and often undetected way.

Dengue virus infection in humans of all four virus serotypes causes a spectrum of illness ranging from inapparent or mild febrile illness to severe and fatal haemorrhagic disease (WHO, 1986). Clinical presentation in both children and adults may vary in severity, but in dengue-endemic areas, acute dengue infections are often clinically non-specific, especially in children, with signs and symptoms of a viral syndrome. The differential diagnosis includes measles, rubella, influenza, typhoid, leptospirosis, malaria and other viral, bacterial and parasitic diseases that cause a dengue-like illness.

Classic dengue fever is primarily a disease of older children and adults, is generally self-limiting and rarely fatal. DHF, the severe and potentially fatal form of dengue infection, is primarily a disease of children under the age of 15 years, although it may occur in older children and adults. DHF can be a very dramatic disease: the patient's condition can deteriorate very rapidly, with onset of shock and death. Risk factors for developing severe haemorrhagic disease are not fully understood but include the strain and serotype of the infecting dengue virus, and the immune status, age and genetic background of the patient.

Changing epidemiology of dengue

Dengue fever and *Ae. aegypti* mosquitoes have a worldwide distribution in tropical areas of the world; over 2.5 billion people live in areas of risk (Figure 9.1) (Halstead, 1980; Rosen, 1982; Gubler and Trent, 1994). In 1997, DEN/DHF is the

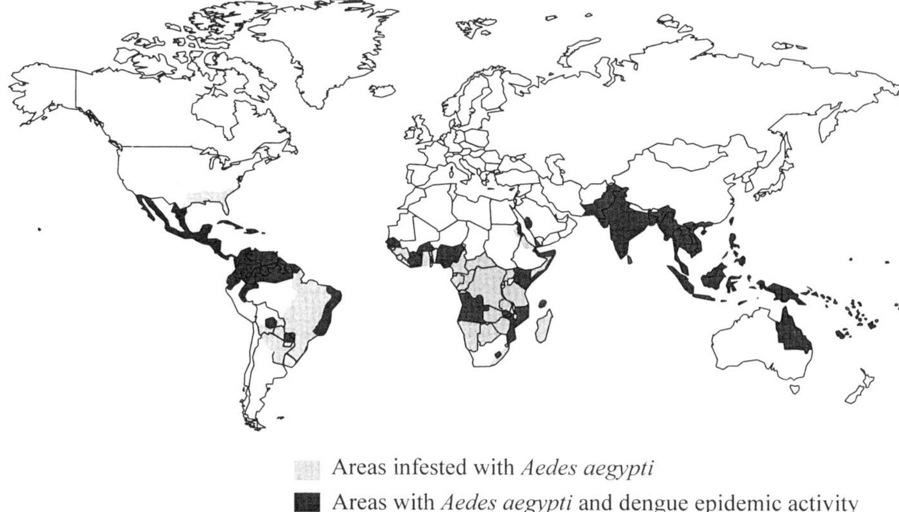

Figure 9.1 The world distribution of epidemic dengue and the principal vector mosquito, *Aedes aegypti*, 1997

most important arboviral disease of humans, with an estimated 50–100 million cases of dengue fever and several hundred thousand cases of DHF occurring each year, depending on epidemic activity (Gubler and Trent, 1994; Monath, 1994; Gubler and Clark, 1995). DHF is a leading cause of hospitalization and death among children in many south-east Asian countries where epidemics first occurred in the 1950s (WHO, 1986). Epidemic DHF has now spread to the South Pacific and the Americas. The pattern of severe haemorrhagic disease evolved in the American region in the 1980s and 1990s similarly to the way it did in south-east Asia in the 1960s and 1970s (Gubler, 1987; 1993). In Central and South America, dengue fever currently has an economic impact of the same order of magnitude as malaria, tuberculosis, sexually transmitted diseases (excluding AIDS), hepatitis, the childhood cluster (polio, measles, pertussis, diphtheria) and the tropical cluster (schistosomiasis, filariasis, Chagas disease, leishmaniasis and onchocerciasis) (Meltzer *et al*, 1997).

The global epidemiology of dengue viruses first began to change with the ecological disruption in south-east Asia during and following World War II (Gubler, 1988; Halstead, 1992). During the war, existing water systems were destroyed, and water storage was increased for domestic use as well as for fire control. War equipment was moved frequently between cities and countries, and large amounts were also left behind. This material collected rainwater and, along with water-storage containers, made ideal larval habitats for the principal vector mosquito, *Ae. aegypti*. The movement of war materials resulted in the transport of mosquitoes and their eggs to new geographical areas. The result of these ecological changes was a greatly expanded geographical distribution and increased population densities of *Ae. aegypti.* In addition, hundreds of thousands of Japanese and Allied soldiers, most of them susceptible to dengue virus infection, were constantly transferred between countries in Asia and the Pacific. This provided a mechanism for movement of dengue viruses between cities, countries and other regions, as well for providing susceptible individuals for epidemic transmission. The war years were thus responsible for creating the conditions (hyperendemicity and high densities of *Ae. aegypti*) for the emergence of DHF in south-east Asia.

In the years following World War II, the unprecedented urbanization of south-east Asia began, with millions of people moving to the cities of the region. Urban centres in most countries expanded rapidly in an uncontrolled and unplanned fashion. Housing was inadequate for large numbers of people, and water, sewer and waste management systems deteriorated. The *Ae. aegypti* populations and dengue viruses thrived in this new ecological setting, with increased transmission and increased frequency of dengue epidemics occurring in the indigenous children, as the adult populations became immune to the viruses. Moreover, an economic expansion in the region began and continues today. This led to continued urbanization and increased movement of people (and with them, dengue viruses) between cities and countries. Those countries that did not already have multiple virus serotypes co-circulating, quickly became hyperendemic. The viruses, often all four serotypes, were maintained in a human–*Ae. aegypti*–human cycle in most urban centres of south-east Asia. The results of these changes were dramatically increased dengue transmission and the emergence of DHF. In every country where the disease emerged as a major public health problem it evolved in a similar manner, first as sporadic cases of DHF occurring for several years, ultimately culminating in a major epidemic. Following the first epidemic, a pattern of epidemic activity was established, with epidemics occurring every three to five years. Characteristically, succeeding epidemics became progressively larger as a result of geographic expansion of DHF within the country.

From the mid-1950s to the 1970s, epidemic DHF was localised in a few south-east Asian countries. The 1980s and 1990s saw a dramatic geographic expansion of epidemic DHF, west into India, Pakistan, Sri Lanka and the Maldive Islands and east into the People's Republic of China (Figure 9.2). There was also a resurgence of disease in Singapore, which had effectively controlled DHF for nearly 20 years; in 1996, Singapore experienced its largest outbreak in history.

Surveillance for DHF is passive in most dengue-endemic countries. Physicians are relied upon to report disease to the health ministry and, typically, only severe cases are reported to the World Health Organization. Thus, only the tip of the iceberg is reported, making DEN/DHF one of the most under-reported tropical infectious diseases in the past 20 years. Even so, approximately four times as

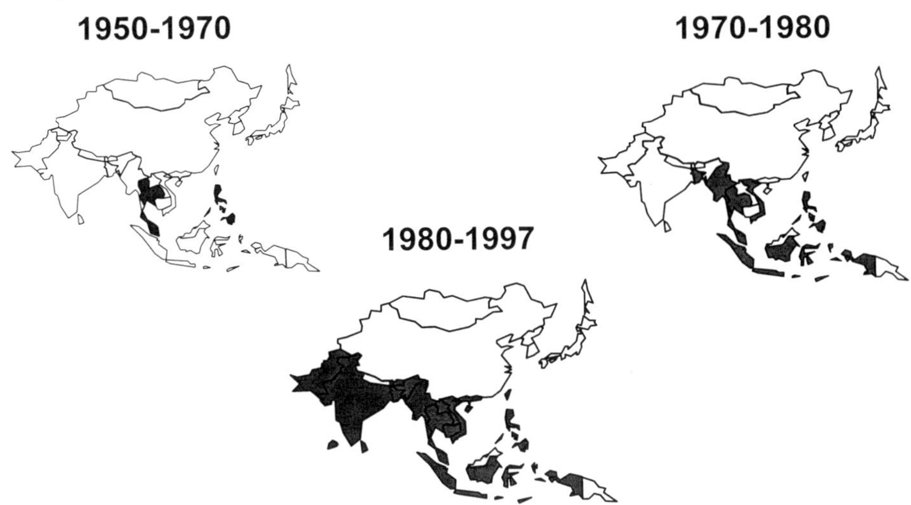

Figure 9.2 The geographic expansion of epidemic dengue haemorrhagic fever in Asia, 1950–1997

many DHF cases have been reported in the past 15 years (1981–95) as in the previous 30 years.

Epidemic dengue re-emerged as a public health problem in the Americas in the late 1970s after a 40-year quiescence, which was due to an *Ae. aegypti* eradication programme initiated by the Pan American Health Organization (PAHO) in 1946 to prevent urban epidemics of yellow fever (Soper *et al*, 1943; Schliessman and Calheiros, 1974). The programme was successful and eradication was achieved in most countries of the region. Unfortunately, the programme was discontinued in the early 1970s, and failure to eradicate *Ae. aegypti* from all countries of the region resulted in repeated reinfestations by this mosquito of those countries that had achieved eradication. During the 1970s, support for *Ae. aegypti* surveillance and control programmes waned, and they were merged with malaria control programmes in many countries. By the end of the 1980s, *Ae. aegypti* had reinfested much of the area from which it had been eradicated in the 1950s and 1960s (PAHO, 1979; Gubler, 1988; 1989). The reinfestation of the region has continued during the 1990s, and in 1997, *Ae. aegypti* has a distribution similar to that in the 1940s, before eradication was initiated.

The expanding geographic distribution of *Ae. aegypti* in the Americas during the 1970s and 1980s coincided with increased movement of dengue viruses both into and within the region (Gubler, 1987; 1993). Prior to 1977, only DEN-2 and DEN-3 viruses were known to be present in the Americas, although DEN-1 was probably present in the early 1940s (Ehrenkranz *et al*, 1971; Gubler, 1987; 1993). A characteristic of dengue in the Americas from the 1950s through to the early

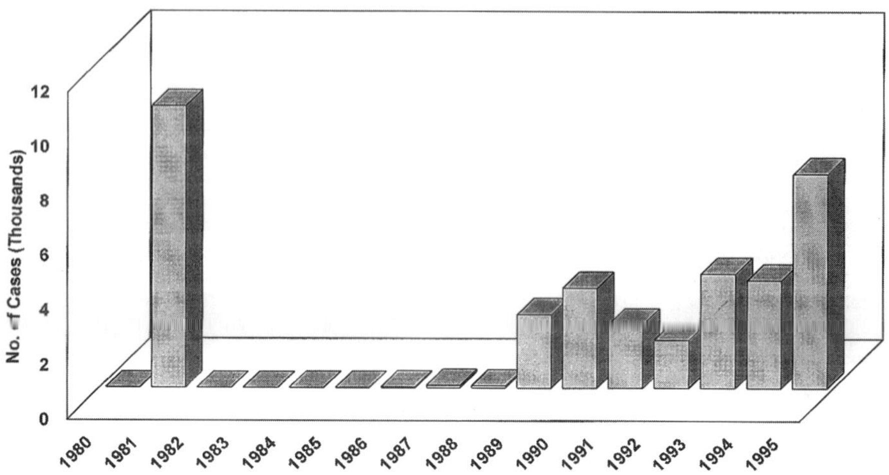

Figure 9.3 The emergence of dengue haemorrhagic fever in the Americas; reported cases to PAHO, 1980–1995. The 1981 figures reflect the Cuban epidemic only

1980s was non-endemicity (no viruses present) or hypoendemicity (only a single serotype present) in a country (Ehrenkranz *et al*, 1971; PAHO, 1979; Gubler, 1987; 1993; 1997).

DEN-1 was reintroduced to the American region in 1977, with epidemics in Jamaica and Cuba; this serotype subsequently spread throughout the Caribbean Islands, Mexico, Texas, Central America and northern South America, causing major or minor epidemics over the next four years (PAHO, 1979; Gubler, 1987; 1993). In 1981, DEN-4 was introduced into the eastern Caribbean Islands and, like DEN-1, this serotype also spread rapidly to other islands in the Caribbean, and to Mexico, Central America and northern South America, causing major or minor epidemics, many of them in countries that had experienced recent DEN-1 epidemics (Gubler, 1987; 1993). Some of these outbreaks (Surinam, 1982; Mexico, 1984; Puerto Rico, 1986; El Salvador, 1987) were associated with the first documented emergence of DHF, which occurred sporadically for the most part (Gubler, 1987; 1993; Kouri *et al*, 1989).

Also in 1981, a new strain of DEN-2 was introduced into Cuba from south-east Asia (Kouri *et al*, 1989; Rico-Hesse, 1990; Lewis *et al*, 1993; Gubler and Trent, 1994). Unlike the DEN-1 and DEN-4 epidemics, the 1981 Cuban DEN-2 epidemic was associated with thousands of cases of severe haemorrhagic disease (Figure 9.3); this was the first major DHF epidemic in the Americas (Kouri *et al*, 1989). Although the viruses isolated in Cuba have been unavailable for study, DEN-2 viruses isolated in Jamaica during and shortly after the Cuban epidemic (Gubler DJ, unpublished data) were sequenced, and the data suggest that the virus causing the epidemic was a new strain introduced from Asia, most likely from Vietnam, where several thousand Cuban aid personnel were working at the time (Rico-Hesse, 1990; Gubler DJ, unpublished data).

The second major epidemic of DHF in the Americas, also thought to be caused by this new strain of DEN-2, occurred in Venezuela in 1989–90 with over 6000 cases and 73 deaths (PAHO, 1990). Epidemic DHF of variable intensity caused by this genotype of DEN-2 subsequently occurred in Colombia (1990), Brazil (1992 and 1994), French Guiana (1992), Puerto Rico (1994) and Mexico (1995), but none of these epidemics was of the same magnitude and severity as the Cuban epidemic of 1981. Other outbreaks involving this genotype of DEN-2 did not cause DHF, even though they had been preceded by DEN-1 and/or DEN-4 outbreaks.

In 1994, a new strain of DEN-3 was introduced into the American region, causing a major epidemic of DEN/DHF in Nicaragua and a small outbreak associated with classical dengue fever in Panama (CDC, 1995). This virus, which was shown to be genetically distinct from the DEN-3 that previously occurred in the Americas (Lanciotti *et al*, 1994; Lanciotti R, Quiros I, Clark GG and Gubler DJ, unpublished data), apparently was also a recent introduction from Asia; it spread throughout Central America and Mexico in 1995, causing major epidemics. Surprisingly, by early 1997 it had yet to be detected in the Caribbean islands or South America.

The sequence of events associated with the changing epidemiology of dengue in the Americas in the 1970s, 1980s and 1990s was nearly identical to that which occurred in south-east Asia in the 1950s, 1960s and 1970s (Gubler, 1987; 1993). Thus, reinvasion of Central and South America by *Ae. aegypti* in the 1970s and 1980s, combined with increased urbanization, increased movement of people and with them, dengue viruses, resulted in most countries evolving from non-endemicity (no viruses present), or hypoendemicity (one virus present) to hyperendemicity (multiple virus serotypes co-circulating). This condition resulted in increased frequency of epidemic activity and the emergence of DHF as a major public health problem. Several countries (Cuba, Venezuela, Brazil and Nicaragua) have had major epidemics of DHF in recent years. Moreover, outbreaks with sporadic or small numbers of cases of DHF have occurred in Nicaragua, Honduras, El Salvador, Guatemala, Mexico, Colombia, French Guiana, Surinam, Aruba, St Lucia and Puerto Rico, and sporadic cases of DHF have been confirmed in the Dominican Republic, the US Virgin Islands, Panama and Costa Rica. In 1980, DHF was not considered endemic in any American country. Between 1981 and 1997, however, there was a dramatic emergence of DHF: 17 countries reported laboratory-confirmed DHF that met the WHO case definition (Figure 9.4). This disease is now endemic in most of those countries where multiple dengue virus serotypes co-circulate, and numbers of the cases reported to PAHO have increased dramatically (Figure 9.3). If the disease pattern continues to evolve in the Americas as it did in south-east Asia, the first 10 years of the 21st century will

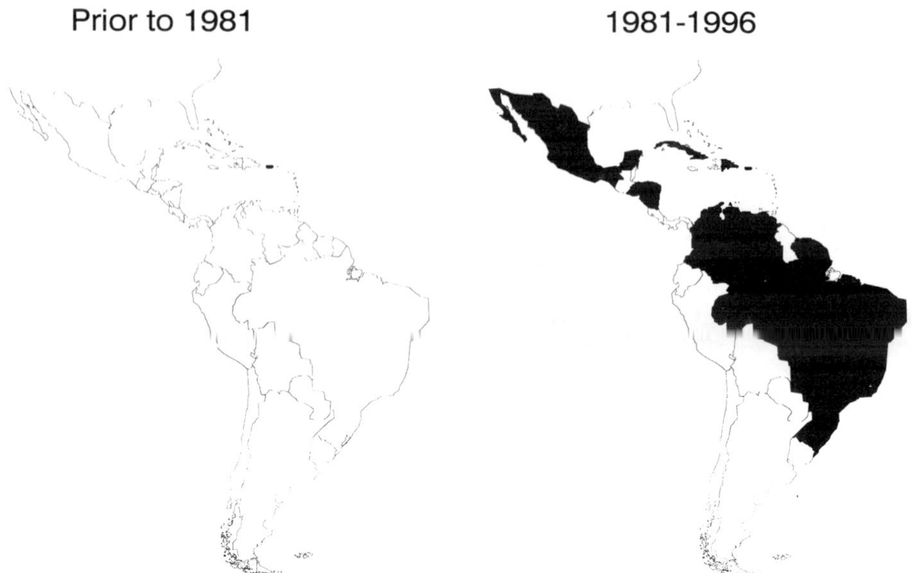

Figure 9.4 Countries with laboratory-confirmed cases of dengue haemorrhagic fever meeting the WHO case definition, prior to 1981, and from 1981 to 1996

bring more frequent and larger epidemics of DHF (Gubler, 1987; 1993).

Surveillance for dengue in Africa has been poor during this century, and epidemics, when they have occurred, were most often initially reported as malaria. Although surveillance has not improved, laboratory-confirmed reports of epidemic dengue fever have increased dramatically since 1980 (Figure 9.5). Limited outbreaks have occurred in West Africa, but the most recent epidemic activity has occurred in East Africa and the Middle East (Gubler, 1997). All four dengue serotypes have been involved, and although sporadic cases of disease clinically compatible with DHF have been reported in some epidemics of dengue fever, DHF in its epidemic form has not yet occurred in Africa or the Middle East.

Factors responsible for the global resurgence of dengue

The reasons for the dramatic resurgence of epidemic DEN/DHF in the waning years of the 20th century are complex and not fully understood, but are most likely associated with demographic and societal changes that have occurred over the past 50 years, as noted above (Gubler and Trent, 1994; Gubler, 1997). The most important demographic changes have been the unprecedented population growth, primarily in tropical developing countries. Coincident with this has been uncontrolled and unplanned urbanization in these same countries. These changes have resulted in large, crowded human populations living in urban centres in substandard housing with inadequate water, sewer and waste management

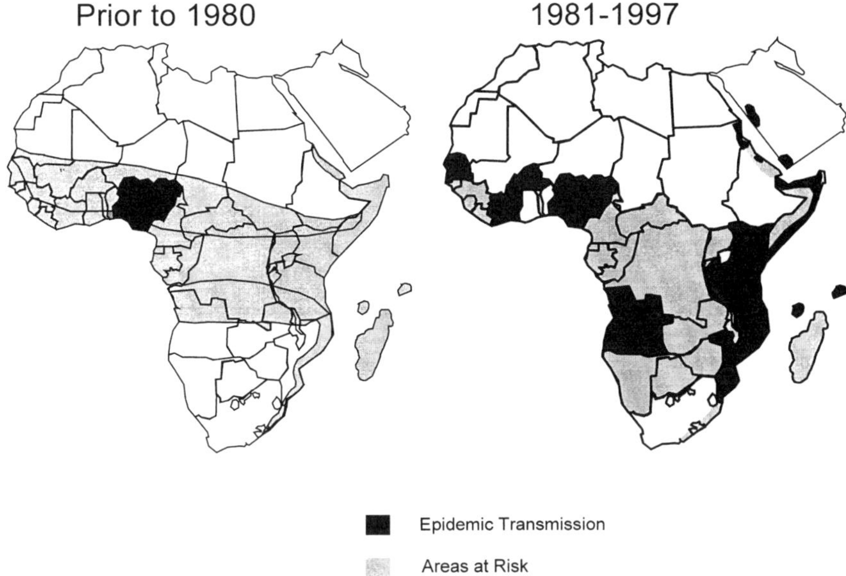

Figure 9.5 Geographic expansion of epidemic dengue fever in Africa and the Middle East, 1980–1997

systems. Most consumer goods are now packaged in non-biodegradable plastic or cellophane which is discarded into the environment, where it collects rainwater and provides ideal larval habitats for the vector mosquito. Also, used car tyres make ideal mosquito larval habitats, and the numbers have increased dramatically in the past 20 years, along with the numbers of cars; tyres are very difficult to dispose of from the environment. All of these factors have contributed to the expanded geographical distribution and increased population densities of the principal mosquito vector, *Ae. aegypti*.

Moreover, the car has increased the mobility of people within and between population centres in a country, enhancing the ability of dengue viruses to spread locally in infected persons or mosquitoes, and thus the development and maintenance of multiple virus serotypes (hyperendemicity) in a country or region. Another contributing factor has been the lack of effective *Ae. aegypti* mosquito control in most dengue-endemic countries of the world. Emphasis for the past 25 years has been placed on ultra-low volume space sprays of insecticide for adult mosquito control (Gubler, 1989). This has been shown to be ineffective in controlling *Ae. aegypti* (Gubler, 1989; Newton and Reiter, 1992). Thus, hundreds of millions of people in urban centres of the tropics are living in intimate association with large populations of an efficient epidemic mosquito vector of dengue viruses, providing ideal conditions for increased transmission of urban mosquito-borne disease such as dengue.

The jet airplane has also had a major impact on the emergence of DEN/DHF. The rapid and efficient movement of people has changed global demographics and has provided the ideal mechanism for dengue viruses to move with ease between countries and continents. The reinfestation of the American tropics by *Ae. aegypti* placed at risk for dengue infection, large numbers of susceptible individuals living in permissive urban areas. The numerous epidemics and increased transmission of dengue that subsequently occurred there, in Asia, the Pacific and Africa, provided increased opportunities for the viruses to move between countries, both within and between the regions, and has resulted in a constant exchange of dengue viruses and other pathogens. An illustration of the increased human air travel is seen in US Department of Transportation data. From 1983 to 1994, the number of international departures from US airports doubled from 20 to nearly 40 million, with over 50% of those departures each year to tropical areas (Gubler, 1996). On a global basis, these numbers would be increased several fold.

Finally, the public health infrastructure required to deal with epidemic vector-borne infectious diseases has deteriorated during the past 30 years in most countries. Limited financial and human resources, and competing priorities for those resources, have resulted in a 'crisis mentality' among public health officials. The emphasis has thus been on implementing emergency control methods in response to epidemics rather than on developing programmes to prevent epidemic transmission (Gubler, 1989). This approach has been particularly detrimental to dengue prevention and control because in most countries surveillance is very poor; the passive surveillance systems relied on to detect increased transmission are dependent upon reports by local physicians, who often have a low index of suspicion for dengue and do not consider it in their differential diagnosis of dengue-like illness. As a result, the epidemic has often reached or passed peak transmission before it is detected and emergency control measures are implemented, always too late to have any impact on the course of the epidemic (Gubler, 1989).

Prospects for the future

There is currently no vaccine for DEN/DHF. Although live, attenuated vaccine candidates for all four virus serotypes have been developed (Bhamarapravati and Yoksan, 1997) it will probably be at least 10 years before they are available for general use. Prospects for reversing the trend of increased epidemic DEN/DHF in the near future must rely on mosquito control and, therefore, are not promising. New dengue virus strains and serotypes will likely continue to move between population centres where *Ae. aegypti* occurs, in infected air travellers, resulting in continued hyperendemicity, increased frequency of epidemic activity and increased incidence of DHF if effective prevention programmes are not implemented without delay. This will require changing the emergency response mentality of government officials, public health professionals and the public, to one of disease prevention.

Effective, sustainable prevention programmes for DEN/DHF must include several components (Gubler and Casta-Valez, 1991). First, an active, laboratory-based surveillance system that can provide early warning for epidemic activity is essential. Health officials in dengue-endemic areas must know at any point in time where dengue transmission is occurring, what serotypes are being transmitted and the severity of illness associated with dengue infection. Moreover, there must be effective use of surveillance data, with information exchange and international cooperation. A second component of an effective prevention programme is a rapid response contingency mosquito control plan to prevent an incipient epidemic when the surveillance system predicts increased dengue transmission. Political support to implement this rapid response in a timely manner is critical to its success. A third component of a sustainable prevention programme is education of the medical community. Experience has shown that case-fatality rates can be kept acceptably low if physicians and nurses understand the pathophysiological changes that occur in DHF; early diagnosis and effective management are the keys to preventing fatalities in this disease (WHO, 1986). A fourth component is community-based, integrated *Ae. aegypti* control. Substainability of the prevention programme will depend on decreasing the reliance on government mosquito control agencies, and the transfer of more responsibility for *Ae. aegypti* control to homeowners in urban areas, where most dengue transmission occurs. This will require community participation and community ownership of the programme. Lastly, there is a great need for research and an improved public health infrastructure. Research is desperately needed to develop more effective prevention strategies, including new mosquito control technology and dengue vaccines, and on the epidemiology and disease pathogenesis of DEN/DHF. Only with an improved public health infrastructure to support community-based prevention programmes will we be able to reverse the trend of emergent epidemic DEN/DHF.

References

Bhamarapravati N, Yoksan S. Live attenuated tetravalent dengue vaccine. In: Gubler DJ, Kuno G (eds), *Dengue and Dengue Hemorrhagic Fever*. London: CAB International Press, 1997, pp 367–377

Centers for Disease Control (CDC). Imported dengue—United States, 1993–1994. *Morbidity and Mortality Weekly Report*, 1995; **44**: 353–356

Ehrenkranz NJ, Ventura AK, Cuadrado RR, Pond WL, Porter JE. Pandemic dengue in Caribbean countries and the southern United States—past, present and potential problems. *New England Journal of Medicine*, 1971; **285**: 1460–1469

Gubler DJ. Dengue and dengue hemorrhagic fever in the Americas. *Puerto Rico Health Sciences Journal*, 1987; **6**: 107–111

Gubler DJ. Dengue. In: Monath TP (ed), *Epidemiology of Arthropod-Borne Viral Disease.*

Boca Raton: CRC Press, 1988, Vol. II, Chapter 23, pp 223–260

Gubler DJ. *Aedes aegypti* and *Aedes aegypti*-borne disease control in the 1990s: top down or bottom up. *American Journal of Tropical Medicine and Hygiene*, 1989; **40**: 571–578

Gubler DJ. Dengue and dengue hemorrhagic fever in the Americas. In: Thoncharoen P (ed), *Dengue Hemorrhagic Fever*. New Delhi, India: World Health Organization, 1993 (WHO Monograph, Reg Pub SEARO No 22) pp 9–22

Gubler DJ. Arboviruses as imported disease agents: the need for increased awareness. *Archives of Virology*, 1996; **11**: 21–32

Gubler DJ. Dengue and dengue hemorrhagic fever: its history and resurgence as a global public health problem. In: Gubler DJ, Kuno G (eds), *Dengue and Dengue Hemorrhagic Fever*. London: CAB International, 1997, pp 1–22

Gubler DJ, Casta-Valez A. A program for prevention and control of epidemic dengue and dengue hemorrhagic fever in Puerto Rico and the U.S. Virgin Islands. *Bulletin of the Pan American Health Organization*, 1991; **25**: 237–247

Gubler DJ, Clark GG. Dengue/Dengue Hemorrhagic Fever: the emergence of a global health problem. *Emerging Infectious Diseases*, 1995; **1**: 55–57

Gubler DJ, Trent DW. Emergence of epidemic dengue/dengue hemorrhagic fever as a public health problem in the Americas. *Infectious Agents and Disease*, 1994; **2**: 383–393

Halstead SB. Dengue hemorrhagic fever—a public health problem and a field for research. *Bulletin of the World Health Organization*, 1980; **58**: 1–21

Halstead SB. The XXth century dengue pandemic: need for surveillance and research. *World Health Statistics Quarterly*, 1992; **45**: 292–329

Knudsen AB, Sloof R. Vector-borne disease problems in rapid urbanization: new approaches to vector control. *Bulletin of the World Health Organization*,1992; **70**: 1–6

Kouri GP, Guzman MG, Bravo JR, Triana C. Dengue haemorrhagic fever/dengue shock syndrome: lessons from the Cuban epidemic, 1981. *Bulletin of the World Health Organization*, 1989; **67**: 375–380

Lanciotti RS, Lewis JG, Gubler DJ, Trent DW. Molecular evolution and epidemiology of dengue-3 viruses. *Journal of General Virology*, 1994; **75**: 65–75

Lewis JA, Chang GJ, Lanciotti RS, Kinney RM, Mayer LW, Trent DW. Phylogenetic relationships of dengue-2 viruses. *Virology*, 1993; **197**: 216–224

Meltzer MI, Rigau-Perez JG, Clark GG, Reiter R, Gubler DJ. Using DALYs to assess the economic impact of dengue in Puerto Rico: 1984–1994. *American Journal of Tropical Medicine and Hygiene*, 1997; in press

Monath TP. Dengue: the risk to developed and developing countries. *Proceedings of the National Academy of Sciences of the USA*, 1994; **91**: 2395–2400

Newton EAC, Reiter P. A model of the transmission of dengue fever with an evaluation of the impact of ultra-low volume (ULV) insecticide applications on dengue epidemics. *American Journal of Tropical Medicine & Hygiene*, 1992; **47**: 709–720

Pan American Health Organization (PAHO). *Dengue in the Caribbean, 1977. Proceedings of a Workshop Held in Montego Bay, Jamaica, 8–11 May, 1978*. PAHO Science Publication 375, 1979

Pan American Health Organization (PAHO). Dengue hemorrhagic fever in Venezuela. *Epidemiological Bulletin*, 1990; **11**: 7–9

Plant AE. *Infecting Ourselves: How Environmental and Social Disruptions Trigger Disease*. Washington, DC: Worldwatch Institute, 1996, Worldwatch paper no 129

Rico-Hesse R. Molecular evolution and distribution of dengue viruses type 1 and 2 in nature. *Virology*, 1990; **174**: 479–493

Rosen L. Dengue—An overview. In: Mackenzie JS (ed), *Viral Diseases in South-East Asia and the Western Pacific*. Sydney: Academic Press, 1982, pp 484–493

Schliessman DJ, Calheiros LB. A review of the status of yellow fever and *Aedes aegypti*

eradication programs in the Americas. *Mosquito News*, 1974; **34**: 1–9
Soper FL, Wilson DB, Lima S, Antunes WS. *The Organization of Permanent Nationwide Anti-*Aedes aegypti *Measure in Brazil.* New York: The Rockefeller Foundation, 1943
World Health Organization (WHO). Dengue haemorrhagic fever: diagnosis, treatment and control. Geneva: World Health Organization, 1986
World Resources Institute, United Nations Environment Programme, United Nations Development Programme, World Bank. *World Resources—1996–1997.* New York: Oxford University Press, 1996

10
BSE and CJD

Peter G. Smith

Department of Infectious and Tropical Diseases, London School of Hygiene & Tropical Medicine, UK

Whether the recently described new variant of Creutzfeldt–Jakob disease (CJD) will command a chapter or a footnote in the history of public health remains to be seen. The first 10 cases of this condition were reported just over a year ago (Will *et al*, 1996). Since that time a further seven cases have been recognized—six in the UK and one in France (Chazot *et al*, 1996). However, there is no doubt that the epidemic of bovine spongiform encephalopathy (BSE) that has affected UK cattle over the past 15 years will deserve a chapter in the history of animal health. To date over 166 000 cases of BSE have been diagnosed, and it is likely that over a million cattle have been infected with the causative agent (Anderson *et al*, 1996)—most of them having been slaughtered and eaten before they had time to show clinical signs of disease.

This chapter reviews the events leading up to the announcement in April 1996 that a new variant of CJD (nvCJD) had emerged and that the most probable explanation for this was infection of humans with the agent responsible for the epidemic of BSE in cattle. The chapter summarizes the evidence for a causative link between nvCJD and BSE available at that time and the extent to which the strength of that evidence has changed in the past year.

When the announcement of the new variant cases was first made it followed a cluster of deaths in the first few months of 1996, and there were fears that a rapid rise in the number of cases of the disease might be seen in the following months. As there have been only six new cases in the past year in the UK, some have questioned whether or not a large epidemic is likely to occur. It is still too early to tell, but I describe some work done with colleagues at the London School of Hygiene & Tropical Medicine and the National CJD Surveillance Unit to explore how informative the numbers of cases arising in the next few years might be in aiding predictions of the eventual size of the epidemic.

New and Resurgent Infections: Prediction, Detection and Management of Tomorrow's Epidemics.
Edited by B. Greenwood and K. De Cock.

The BSE epidemic

The first confirmed case of BSE in cattle was diagnosed in 1986 and since then there have been nearly 167 000 confirmed cases. The epidemic peaked with over 3000 cases per month at the end of 1992 and since then has been steadily declining to fewer than 500 cases per month by 1997, though the decline has not been at the rate that had been originally hoped. None the less, it is expected that by the turn of the century the epidemic in cattle will be virtually over (Anderson *et al*, 1996).

In 1987, BSE was thought to be a new disease of cattle, and it was soon recognised that early cases might herald a major epidemic. Early in the epidemic, Wilesmith and colleagues at the Central Veterinary Laboratories investigated various hypotheses to explain the start of the epidemic (Wilesmith *et al*, 1991). The key risk factor identified was the use of commercial concentrate feed and, in particular, the feeding of meat and bone meal to calves.This focused attention on changes that had taken place in rendering processes in the early 1980s which might have correlated with the onset of the epidemic, if the disease had an average incubation period of four to five years.

For several decades the waste tissues of cattle and sheep that were not used for other purposes were rendered (essentially a boiling and fat extraction process) and used to make meat and bone meal. This was used as a protein-rich dietary supplement for cattle and other farmed animals. The introduction of this practice long preceded the start of the BSE epidemic, but the onset of the epidemic was found to correlate with changes that had been made in the rendering processes on a widespread basis in the early 1980s. In particular, the use of a solvent fat extraction process was stopped and a 'live steam stripping' process to recover solvent was consequently eliminated. It is thought that these two changes may have been sufficient to allow the causative agent of BSE to survive the rendering process.

The favoured hypothesis for the origin of the agent is that it derives from a strain of scrapie, a transmissible spongiform encephalopathy which is endemic in British sheep. It is supposed that this strain crossed from sheep to cattle through the rendering of scrapie-infected waste sheep tissues. The scrapie agent was then consumed by cattle in meat and bone meal and the strain became adapted to the cattle population. An alternative hypothesis is that BSE had previously been endemic in cattle at a very low level but had not been detected and that changes in the rendering processes allowed it to be recycled and spread in cattle through contaminated meat and bone meal (Spongiform Encephalopathy Advisory Committee, 1995).

At present, it is not known which of these hypotheses, if either, is true. To date no strain of scrapie has been found in the sheep population which appears to be the same as BSE, but only limited strain typing of scrapie has been done (Bruce, 1993) and it possible that strain characteristics changed as the species barrier was crossed.

The epidemic of BSE has been confined almost completely to the UK, with only a few cases reported from European and other countries—mostly associated with the export of cattle or feed from the UK. Why the epidemic occurred in the UK and not elsewhere is not clear, but it may be significant that the sheep-to-cattle ratio in the UK is much higher than in most other countries in which scrapie is endemic.

Once the probable mode of transmission of the BSE agent was identified a ban was placed on the feeding of ruminant protein to ruminants in July 1988. This measure was expected to stop transmission and it was predicted that the total size of the epidemic would be between 17 000 and 20 000 cases (Working Party on Bovine Spongiform Encephalopathy, 1989). In fact this early estimate was out by an order of magnitude and there have now been 166 000 cases. There are two principal reasons that the early estimate was in error. First, insufficient account was taken of the recycling of infected material once the disease was in the cattle population; further transmission then involved no crossing of a species barrier. Secondly, there were various deficiencies in the application of the feed ban, which caused transmission by the feed route to continue much longer than had been anticipated. Over 32 000 cases of BSE have been recorded in cattle born after the feed ban had been introduced, including a few cases in cattle born as late as 1993.

The ruminant feed ban was the principal measure taken to protect animal health. The principal measure taken to minimise the risk to humans (which risk was considered to be remote) was the specified bovine offals ban, introduced in November 1989. This prohibited certain cattle organs being used for human consumption, the most important being the brain and spinal cord, which were the only tissues shown to have evidence of infectivity in challenge studies performed in mice and cattle.

New spongiform encephalopathies have been observed in some zoo animals and domestic cats as well as in cattle. Strain typing of the agents responsible for these cases has shown them to have the same characteristics as the BSE agent (Bruce *et al*, 1994) and it is assumed that these animals were infected either through the consumption of the same meat and bone meal that was fed to cattle or through the consumption of neural tissue from infected cows, either as raw meat or in cat food.

The link with CJD

Initially, it was considered most unlikely that BSE would have any implications for human health (Working Party on Bovine Spongiform Encephalopathy, 1989), principally because the favoured hypothesis for the origin of the BSE agent was that it was derived from the agent responsible for scrapie in sheep and it was known that sheep had been infected with this agent for over 200 years without any evidence of harm to humans. However, as a precautionary measure, a national CJD Surveillance Unit was established in 1990 to monitor any changes in the incidence of the disease that might indicate that BSE had infected the human population. It was not clear exactly what clinical features might be associated with such infection, but it was thought that if such infection *did* occur, the disease caused would most likely resemble CJD.

There had been a previous attempt to identify all cases of CJD in England and Wales from 1970 onwards and in the UK as a whole from 1985 onwards. Because there are only about 100 neurologists in the UK it was possible to liaise directly with them and with neuropathologists to ascertain cases, though checks were also made on death certificates for additional cases. A prospective surveillance system had been set up for cases occurring between 1980 and 1984 in England and Wales and cases were also ascertained retrospectively for the period 1970–79. Following the setting up of the National CJD Surveillance Unit in 1990, cases occurring in the UK between 1985 and 1989 were also ascertained retrospectively.

From 1970 to the mid-1990s the number of confirmed cases of CJD in England and Wales rose from about 10 a year to around 40 per year. The pattern of increase did not correspond well with that of the BSE epidemic and it was thought most likely that the increase was due to enhanced ascertainment of cases and that it did not represent a true increase in the incidence of the disease. Evidence in support of this was the fact that the largest increase was in persons over the age of 70 years, subjects in whom other causes of dementia are relatively common and in whom only a small proportion of deaths would be followed by autopsy examination (Cousens *et al*, 1997b). The incidence of CJD is extremely low below the age of 50 years, after which it rises to a peak of about 2/million/year in the 60–69-year age group, thereafter declining rapidly (Will *et al*, 1986). There has been speculation about the reason for this decline in old age, but a favoured explanation for at least part of the decline is poor ascertainment of cases in old people.

In 1995, an excess risk of CJD was reported among cattle farmers in the UK, a group likely to be at increased risk of exposure to the BSE agent, but this finding was difficult to interpret as a similar increase was found among cattle farmers in other European countries where there had been few cases of BSE (Cousens *et al*, 1997b).

The first real indications that the epidemiology of CJD in the UK might be changing came in 1995 when two cases of CJD were reported among teenagers; by March 1996 it was clear that the age distribution of the disease was changing. In the 25 years 1970–94 only one case of CJD had been diagnosed in the UK in a patient under the age of 30 years (excluding familial and iatrogenic cases), but during 1995 and the first few months of 1996, six such cases were diagnosed. Statistically, this was extremely unlikely to be a chance occurrence, but the critical additional finding was that the young cases diagnosed in 1995 and 1996 all had a distinctive neuropathology, which had not been seen previously in any of the 175 cases of CJD investigated by the CJD Surveillance Unit. Also, as far as could be ascertained at that time, the neuropathological profile of the cases has

Table 10.1 Basis of 'causative' link between BSE and nvCJD in March 1996

- Geographical limitation of nvCJD and BSE to UK
- Temporal occurrence of nvCJD consistent with incubation period 5–10 years after BSE exposure
- Biologically plausible
- No other persuasive explanation

not been described in cases outside the UK (Will *et al*, 1996).

Faced with this evidence the Spongiform Encephalopathy Advisory Committee, which had been set up to advise the British government on public health issues related to BSE, decided there was good evidence of the emergence of a new variant of CJD in the UK population and that the most likely explanation was that it was due to human infection with the BSE agent. The relatives of new cases of CJD had been questioned about possible dietary and other risk factors for CJD since surveillance started in 1990 and their responses were compared to those of controls. However, no marked differences in dietary habits or other possible risk factors were found between the two groups. The evidence to support a causative link between the BSE agent and nvCJD at that time (March 1996) is summarized in Table 10.1. In the scientific community, opinion varied considerably as to whether or not the link was likely to be a causative one.

During the year since 1996 the evidence for a causal link has strengthened, though is not proven (but short of experimental inoculation of the BSE agent into a human, it is difficult to imagine what would constitute formal 'proof'). The additional evidence that has been acquired is summarised in Table 10.2.

Although nvCJD was thought to be a new disease and restricted to the UK, it was difficult to be sure of this in March 1996 before the characteristic features of the disease were published. However, if cases had occurred in other countries, it would seem reasonable to expect some of these to have been reported by now. Thus, the spatial and temporal evidence in favour of a link between CJD and BSE has been strengthened. Given that substantial numbers of cattle and beef products were exported to France in the 1980s, the occurrence of a single case of nvCJD in France does not seriously challenge the hypothesis of a causative link. Support for the hypothesis was provided by the observation that when BSE-infected tissue was inoculated into the brains of macaques, the neuropathology of the disease that developed was identical to that seen in nvCJD (Lasmezas *et al*, 1996).

The strain typing methods which were first developed to identify different strains of scrapie have so far not identified any strain variation in BSE (Bruce, 1993). It was by the use of these methods that it was shown that the BSE agent was likely to be responsible for the new TSEs seen in some zoo animals and domestic cats. These strain typing methods involve the inoculation of infective tissue into the brains of different strains of mice and subsequent comparison of the incubation periods and neuropathology of the disease when it develops. Such studies have been set up for nvCJD but, because they involve injecting infected

Table 10.2 Supportive evidence for causative link in year following March 1996

- No cases of nvCJD found with onset before 1994
- Only one case described outside the UK (France)
- Similar pathology when BSE injected into macaque
- Strain-typing studies

tissue into mouse brain and waiting for disease to develop, these studies take over a year to complete and the first results are not expected until later in 1997.

However, a new biochemical method of characterizing different possible strains, which can be conducted much more rapidly than the method based on mouse inoculation, has given results which support a causal link between BSE and nvCJD. Collinge *et al* (1996) showed that in their test system, which examines the patterns of protease-resistant prion protein (PrP) on Western blots, nvCJD was distinctly different from other forms of CJD. However, the Western blot pattern of nvCJD closely resembled that obtained using neural tissue of two strains of mice, a macaque and a cat, all of which were infected or, in the case of the cat, presumed to be infected, with BSE. The original paper by Collinge and colleagues contained no data on sheep scrapie strains. A recently published paper (Parchi *et al*, 1997) reported similar analysis on scrapie strains passaged through mice; BSE could not be distinguished from at least one scrapie strain. Experience with this new strain typing system is limited and although the results available are quite strongly suggestive of a causal link between BSE and nvCJD, they are not conclusive. More definitive data will become available later in 1997 when results from the more established mouse-model strain typing system become available.

How the human epidemic might evolve

If a causal link between the BSE agent and nvCJD is accepted, is it possible now to say how many people will eventually be infected? If it is too soon to do this, how soon might we be able to make predictions with more confidence? We have explored some simple mathematical models to begin to address these questions (Cousens *et al*, 1997a), but we fully recognise that any conclusions at this stage must be very tentative, as extrapolations are based on only the 16 cases of nvCJD that have been diagnosed in the UK to date.

The models developed are based upon the assumption that the number of cases arising in a given year depends upon:

- how many people have been infected,
- when they were infected
- what the distribution of the incubation period is.

At present we know only the number of cases per year for the past few years. In order to estimate how many cases there might be in total we have to make

Table 10.3 Predicted numbers of nvCJD cases assuming lognormal incubation period (assuming ban on specified bovine offals 90% effective)

Mean incubation period (years)	90th centile of incubation period distribution (years)	Predicted cases with onset: pre-1994	in 1996	in 1997	in 1998	Total number of human infections
10	15.0	3	12	15	18	213
	20.0	13	8	8	7	104
15	22.5	1	19	32	48	1 595
	30.0	10	8	9	10	174
20	30.0	1	26	54	97	12 000
	40.0	8	9	10	11	284
25	37.5	1	32	79	166	80 000
	50.0	7	10	11	13	450

assumptions about when infection occurred and what the distribution of incubation periods will be. The details of the approach we have adopted are described elsewhere (Cousens *et al*, 1997a). In brief, we assumed that the number of persons infected each year was directly proportional to the number of BSE cases diagnosed in that year, up until 1989 when the order banning specified offals (including brain and spinal cord) from human consumption was introduced. For subsequent years we assumed that the order was either completely effective (probably optimistically) or was only 90% effective (hopefully, pessimistically). We further assumed that the distribution of incubation periods might be one of three mathematical distributions (lognormal, Weibull or Gamma), which are commonly used to model infectious diseases, with mean incubation periods of 5, 10, 15, 20 or 25 years and with 90% of cases arising before 1.5 or 2 times the incubation period. We further constrained the modelling to predict 13 cases with onset in 1994–95, which is the current observed number.

Table 10.3 shows a sample output from the modelling; more extensive results are given elsewhere (Cousens *et al*, 1997a). Each line of the table shows a different possible scenario. Some scenarios can be ruled out with some confidence now (e.g. those which predict substantial numbers of cases with onset prior to 1994—as to date we know of no such cases), but a wide range of other possibilities, compatible with what has been observed to date, remain, ranging from 100 cases or less to many thousands. (It should be noted that the dates in the table relate to the dates of onset. These are usually not ascertained by the CJD Unit until the case is reported to them, which may be a year or more later, so that we may still identify cases which had an onset in 1996.)

Considering all the results from this modelling, we have drawn some tentative conclusions. First, it is premature to conclude that because only 16 cases of nvCJD have been confirmed in the UK to date any subsequent epidemic will necessarily be small. Secondly, the number of cases over the next few years should

Table 10.4 Predicted numbers of nvCJD cases under two different scenarios (assuming ban on specified bovine offals 90% effective)

Mean incubation period (shape of distribution)	90th centile of incubation period distribution (years)	Predicted cases with onset:				Total number of human infections
		pre-1994	in 1996	in 1997	in 1998	
15 years (lognormal)	22.5	1	19	32	48	1 595
25 years (gamma)	37.5	2	18	31	50	13 000

provide a better indication of how large any epidemic might eventually be. Thirdly, if the number of cases with onset in each of the next three years is roughly constant and less than about 20 a year, the final size of the epidemic may well be a few hundred cases or less. Fourthly, if there are 25 or more cases with onset in 1996, with a doubling or tripling in each of the following two years, this would be compatible with a long mean incubation period and an epidemic of many thousands of cases. Fifthly, some possible courses for the epidemic may lead to substantial uncertainty even in three or four years' time. For example, Table 10.4 shows two scenarios with similar findings up to 1998, but which predict epidemics which are an order of magnitude different in size. It must be emphasised that these conclusions are tentative because they are founded on a large number of assumptions, which, though plausible, cannot yet be verified.

Evidence is likely to emerge in the next year which will establish with more confidence whether or not the cases of nvCJD are due to exposure to the BSE agent, but forecasting the future course of the epidemic at this time is still surrounded by areas of great uncertainty and this is likely to remain the case for the immediate future.

References

Anderson RM, Donnelly CA, Ferguson NM *et al.* Transmission dynamics and epidemiology of BSE in British cattle. *Nature*, 1996; **382**: 779–788

Bruce ME. Scrapie strain variation and mutation. *British Medical Bulletin*, 1993; **49**: 822–838

Bruce M, Chree A, McConnell I, Foster J, Pearson G, Fraser H. Transmission of bovine spongiform encephalopathy and scrapie to mice: strain variation and the species barrier. *Philosophical Transactions of the Royal Society of London, Series B: Biological Sciences (London)*, 1994; **343**: 405–411

Chazot G, Broussolle E, Lapras Cl, Blattler T, Aguzzi A, Kopp N. New variant of Creutzfeldt–Jakob disease in a 26-year-old French man. *Lancet*, 1996; **347**: 1181

Collinge J, Sidle KC, Meads J, Ironside J, Hill AF. Molecular analysis of prion strain variation and the aetiology of 'new variant' CJD. *Nature*, 1996; **383**: 685–690

Cousens SN, Vynnycky E, Zeidler M, Will RG, Smith PG. Predicting the CJD epidemic. *Nature*, 1997a; **385**: 197–198

Cousens SN, Zeidler M, Esmonde TF *et al.* Sporadic Creutzfeldt–Jakob disease in the

United Kingdom: epidemiological data from 1970–1996. *British Medical Journal*, 1997b; **315**: 389–394

Lasmezas CI, Deslys J-P, Demalmay R *et al.* BSE transmission to macaques. *Nature*, 1996; **381**: 743–744

Parchi P, Capellari S, Chen SG *et al.* Typing prion isoforms. *Nature*, 1997; **386**: 232–233

Spongiform Encephalopathy Advisory Committee. *Transmissible Spongiform Encephalopathies: A Summary of Present Knowledge and Research.* London: HMSO, 1995

Wilesmith JW, Ryan JB, Atkinson MJ. Bovine spongiform encephalopathy: epidemiological studies on the origin. *The Veterinary Record*, 1991; **128**: 199–203

Will RG, Matthews WB, Smith PG, Hudson C. A retrospective study of Creutzfeldt–Jakob disease in England and Wales 1970–1979. II: Epidemiology. *Journal of Neurology, Neurosurgery and Psychiatry*, 1986; **49**: 749–755

Will RG, Ironside JW, Zeidler M *et al.* A new variant of Creutzfeldt–Jakob disease in the UK. *Lancet*, 1996; **347**: 921–925

Working Party on Bovine Spongiform Encephalopathy. *Report of the Working Party on Bovine Spongiform Encephalopathy.* London: Department of Health and Ministry of Agriculture, Fisheries and Food, 1989

11
Food poisoning

Stephen Palmer

Welsh Combined Centres for Public Health, University of Wales College of Medicine, Cardiff, Wales

The increasing concern over food safety in Western countries highlights a paradox. Although there is a perception amongst the public and media that food is less safe than it used to be, epidemiological evidence suggests the reverse. As serious infections are now relatively rare, the trigger for public alarm has become much more sensitive. Over the past generation, one of the great improvements in the public's health has been the virtual disappearance of typhoid and paratyphoid fevers, bovine tuberculosis and brucellosis, which were primarily food-borne infections, and life-threatening. The common food-borne diseases which have been identified in recent years—non-typhoid salmonellas, campylobacter, SRSV (small round structured viruses)—usually cause only mild self-limiting gastroenteritis. Public concern, however, has grown and has recently rightly been fuelled by the emergence of verotoxigenic *Escherichia coli* (VTEC) and new-variant CJD.

Studies of risk perception (Fischhoff *et al*, 1993) suggest that the public becomes especially alarmed about health threats if the type of death at risk is vivid; exposure is involuntary; exposure is unnatural; there is lack of personal experience of the risk; the effects of exposure are delayed; they do not trust the control agencies; and highly valued institutions are threatened.

Public concern is mediated by newspaper, television and radio so that factors which make health issues into media health scares must take into account newsworthiness (de Semir, 1996). Factors contributing to newsworthiness include: closeness of event to readers, novelty, seriousness, potential for epidemic, bizarre events, outrage, conflict and blame, cover-up and corruption, and human interest and drama.

In the following examples an attempt is made to distinguish the different contributory factors which have led to the emergence of the particular problem. They will be seen to include both biological and social factors (Table 11.1).

New and Resurgent Infections: Prediction, Detection and Management of Tomorrow's Epidemics.
Edited by B. Greenwood and K. De Cock.

Table 11.1 Causes of epidemics

Organism	Underlying causes	Result
Salmonella enteritidis pt4	Limited genetic stock Oviduct infection Raw egg recipes	All industry affected International epidemic
E. coli O157	Changes in husbandry? Increased movement of cattle? Mass processing of meat? Fast food? New laboratory methods	Better ascertainment Increased incidence
Cryptosporidium	AIDS New laboratory methods	Better ascertainment
Listeria	Mass production International trade in exotic foods	International outbreaks Soft cheese outbreaks
Campylobacter	New laboratory methods New reservoirs	Better ascertainment Magpie/milk outbreaks
SRVS (small round smooth viruses)	Sewage pollution of fisheries Consumption of raw shellfish	Dispersed outbreaks

Salmonella enteritidis pt4 (Se4)

Since the end of the 1980s, Se4 has become epidemic internationally following entry of the infection into the elite breeding flocks of poultry which produce and supply most commercial broilers and layers (GB Advisory Committee on the Microbiological Safety of Food, 1993). The new biological factor involved in this process seems to have been the ability of Se4 to invade the oviduct so that small numbers of salmonellas are deposited in the albumin of the egg. Because the egg industry has a very steep pyramid of production, with only a small number of companies controlling the elite breeding stock, the whole industry was affected. At the consumer level, Se4 outbreaks due to egg consumption were frequently linked to particular catering practices, such as use of raw egg recipes, and cross-contamination from raw to cooked foods. The image of the cherished British egg as the culprit of food poisoning has not been well received by the public, and there has been resistance to the message that eggs should be thoroughly cooked.

Campylobacter

There has been a steady increase in the incidence of campylobacter infection in the UK since its recognition in the late 1970s, following the development of new culture techniques for routine laboratory use. However, the steady increase that has made campylobacter the commonest food-borne disease in the UK has not been explained. Better ascertainment and reporting of cases must have contributed, but there have also been other significant and surprising factors, such as the growth in urban areas of populations of magpies which raid milk delivered to doorsteps and which may transmit the infection (Southern *et al*, 1990).

E.coli 0157

Reasons for the emergence of VTEC infections are not clear. Factors suggested include changes in husbandry, extensive movement of livestock leading to cross-continent spread of infections, the growth of the fast food industry (VTEC was first recognised in outbreaks associated with fast food beefburgers), the biological properties of VTEC including the low dose required to cause infection, and development of more sophisticated laboratory techniques for diagnosis (Armstrong *et al*, 1996).

Listeria

The epidemic in the UK in 1987–89 which caused considerable public alarm was probably due to consumption of paté imported from one factory in Europe (McLauchlin *et al*, 1991), emphasizing the importance of international trade in the changing face of food-borne disease. Mortality associated with listeria is confined to patients with relative immune deficiencies, but the at-risk population is increasing.

SRSV (small round structured viruses)

Viral gastroenteritis has been recognized since the 1980s. The contribution of food-borne infection to the total morbidity caused by SRSV is not quantified, but outbreaks due to consumption of bivalve molluscs harvested from sewage-polluted beds have led to large national and international outbreaks (Dowell *et al*, 1995). Normal depuration procedures for cleaning bivalves are not effective for viruses, so that attention has focused on reducing the discharge of sewage into coastal waters as the primary means of preventing this infection.

Cryptosporidium

This protozoan parasitic cause of gastroenteritis was recognized as a major health problem due to the AIDS epidemic. In AIDS patients, cryptosporidium causes life-threatening diarrhoea. Subsequent investigations of non-AIDS cases of diarrhoea revealed cryptosporidium to be a common aetiological agent (Public Health Laboratory Service Study Group, 1990). Large dispersed outbreaks due to domestic water contamination, despite normal chlorination procedures, have led to considerable public concern about the safety of the water supply in several industrialized countries where, in the past, it was generally considered to be beyond reproach.

Causes of epidemics

The above examples illustrate the complex causal network resulting in food-borne infection. Without doubt, new biological factors (for example, oviduct infection by Se4, magpie numbers in urban areas, increasing population of relatively immunosuppressed people) have contributed, but commercial, industrial and social factors are at least as important. These include the mass production and global distribution of foods, international travel, changing food preferences, and the decline in knowledge of 'domestic science'.

The role of the media in turning issues into scares also needs to be analysed. The role the media covets as champion of the public, the public's increasing fascination with fear, increased interest in science and poor conceptualization of risk all add to the potential for publicity for outbreaks of food poisoning. Added to this is the decreased trust in government and the developing 'Green' agenda.

Risk communication

As new food-borne diseases or new modes of transmission modes have been identified, government and industry have acted where possible to reduce the risk, and to inform the public about preventive measures. The major problem for public health, however, is not so much acquiring the biomedical knowledge as addressing the gap between the public and scientific perceptions of risk, and failures of risk communication. A scientific view of the public's lack of understanding is revealed as follows:

> Consumers need educating in the perception of hazard and risk. It seems odd that a 1 in 100 risk of being involved in a car accident, or a 1 in 20,000 risk of being involved in an air incident can be accepted but the same level-headedness cannot be brought to the 1 in 2 million chance of suffering from botulism. (Meldrum, 1994)

However, this misses the point now well described by social psychologists, which is that people may well accept a high level of risk from behaviours they choose to engage in for benefits they perceive. However, risk tolerance is much lower when the risk is seen to be uncontrolled by them, confers no benefit, but is rather the result of a perceived inadequacy of mistrusted agencies.

As far as public agencies are concerned, the following should be noted:

> Often, actions are what people most want to know about. People want to know what you are doing to prevent an accident or how you are preparing for the possibility, not how likely you think one is ... Many people perceive mismanagement, incompetence and lack of conscientiousness as the central issues in risk assessment. Explaining what you have done, are doing and plan to do to reduce and manage the risk is at least as important as explaining how small you think it is. (Covelli *et al*, 1988)

Better risk communication by public health agencies requires a new mind set in which openness and honesty, rather than secrecy and defensiveness, are the foremost features.

References

Armstrong GL, Hollingsworth J, Glen Morris Jr J. Emerging food pathogens: *Escherichia coli* 0157:H7 as a model of entry of a new pathogen into the food supply of the developed world. *Epidemiologic Reviews*, 1996; **18**: 29–51

Covelli V, Sandman P, Slovic P. Risk communication, risk statistics and risk companions. In: *A Manual for Plant Managers*. Washington DC: Chemical Manufacturers Association, 1988

de Semir V. What is newsworthy? *Lancet*, 1996; **347**: 1163–1166

Dowell SF, Groves C, Kirkland KB *et al.* A multi-state outbreak of oyster-associated gastroenteritis: implications for interstate tracing of contaminated shellfish. *Journal of Infectious Diseases*, 1995; **171**: 1497–1503

Fischhoff B, Bostrom A, Quadrel MJ. Risk perception and communication. *Annual Review of Public Health*, 1993; **14**: 183–203

Great Britain Advisory Committee on the Microbiological Safety of Food. *Report on Salmonella in Eggs*. London: HMSO, 1993

McLauchlin J, Hall SM, Velani SK, Gilbert RJ. Human listeriosis and paté: a possible association. *British Medical Journal*, 1991; **303**: 773–775

Meldrum KC. Food safety: whose responsibility is it? *Public Health Laboratory Service Microbiology Digest*, 1994; **11**: 194–198

Public Health Laboratory Service Study Group. Cryptosporidiosis in England and Wales: prevalence and clinical and epidemiological features. *British Medical Journal*, 1990; **300**: 774–777

Southern JP, Smith RM, Palmer SR. Bird attack on milk bottles: possible mode of transmission of *Campylobacter jejuni* to man. *Lancet*, 1990; **336**: 1425–1427

12 Co-ordination of international responses to epidemics

Alain Moren

European Programme for Intervention Epidemiology Training, Reseau National de Santé Publique, Paris, France

Many of the epidemic diseases considered in this volume have prompted international responses of various magnitudes and efficacy. Efficient co-ordination has frequently been challenged by the high number of partners involved and by their different motivations, ranging from public health and humanitarian concerns to research interest or political and media considerations. Co-ordination is a very sensitive issue. We all request co-ordination but not everyone is ready to be co-ordinated. To achieve good international co-ordination, we need common goals with complementary rather than competitive roles for the partners involved in the response. A clear division of labour is necessary and this should be supported by agreed standards of performance. In addition, coherence between the different links in the chain of action is required. In certain circumstances, for example the Great Lake crisis, the task facing the international agencies may be very challenging.

On-site co-ordination

An example of good on-site co-ordination is provided by the Ebola haemorrhagic fever epidemic in Kikwit in 1995 during which 317 cases with 245 deaths were reported. In response to this outbreak a major international intervention was launched, which involved 900 persons from Zaire and outside, among them 131 experts from UN agencies, private, public institutions and non-governmental organizations (NGOs), together with 84 journalists from 13 countries including six from Zaire. The estimated cost of this response was US$7.5 million. Soon after the start of the intervention, an international committee for technical and

New and Resurgent Infections: Prediction, Detection and Management of Tomorrow's Epidemics.
Edited by B. Greenwood and K. De Cock.

scientific co-ordination was set up in Kikwit under the dual leadership of the Zairian authorities and WHO. Responsibility for various aspects of the intervention was placed under the supervision of several sub-commissions. As more human and material resources were brought to Kikwit by local agencies and international aid organizations, these were directed to the appropriate sub-commission.

The work carried out by the sub-commission on epidemiology, clinical management, research and laboratory investigation is described by Pierre Rollin and co-authors (this volume, chapter 8), and reflects the high level of commitment of the Centers for Disease Control and Prevention (CDC) from the USA and a good collaboration with NGOs and the Red Cross. It is also worth mentioning the role of the awareness-raising commission which co-ordinated the work of 300 opinion leaders supported by NGOs. Their role was to inform the population of the nature and the mode of transmission of the epidemic. This led to the control of rumours and helped to avoid further panic in the population. It also helped to restore confidence between the population and the health system. In addition, the co-ordination commission on social affairs permitted the reintegration of affected families. Overall, 160 families and more than 700 orphans were taken care of.

A further commission dealt with logistical support, which is always a key component of a good response. The various NGOs involved made major contributions to appropriate renovation of buildings, storage capacity, provision of communication equipment, vehicles, fuel and also to renovation of the electrical supply for the hospital and the town of Kikwit. To facilitate logistical support in emergencies, several NGOs have created kits of material which enable their teams in the field to be totally independent. Immunization kits have been created by Medecins Sans Frontières (MSF) and Save the Children Fund (SCF), and kits developed by MSF provide accommodation and clinical care for up to 500 patients with cholera. Kits of essential drugs have been developed by NGOs and WHO, and other more practical kits such as energy kits and kits providing daily living essentials for operational teams are available. These resources should be made available during major crises. As an example, such material would have been extremely useful during the recent (early 1997) investigation of an outbreak of monkeypox in Zaire which was logistically difficult and dangerous. Finally, the inventory of all such resources should be carried at international level.

Reports on the effectiveness of the Kikwit intervention have been both optimistic and pessimistic. The optimists point to the way in which effective co-ordination was achieved as a result of the confidence that WHO established with its partners. This was based on an attempt to achieve appropriate division of labour and on the occurrence of regular meetings which allowed for continuous improvement in responses to be made. Finally, an excellent evaluation of performance was achieved through several meetings conducted in Kinshasa and Geneva by the different partners. Results of these evaluations are currently being included in an operational guideline developed under the co-ordination of WHO.

Co-ordination at Kikwit was better than that achieved in many similar previous outbreaks, but there is still room for improvement. Too many inexperienced partners were involved, and international experts rotated too rapidly. In addition the drugs and equipment provided were frequently unsuitable. The media coverage was huge and the presence of journalists, even during co-ordination meetings, discouraged many partners from participating in these meetings. It was impossible to avoid the politicization of different contributions and lack of transparency in the management of financial resources.

Four major lessons can be learned from the Kikwit experience. Good co-ordination means skilled and experienced co-ordinators and, in this regard, Kikwit was a positive event. Logistical support is a key issue and it should be provided by experienced partners such as the major NGOs. In Kikwit a clear attempt was made to clarify the division of labour. However, co-ordination was done on an ad hoc basis and it was not based on the implementation of a previously prepared action plan.

Preparedness

Lessons from the Kikwit intervention show that preparedness is an important step in achieving efficiency. Several components of preparedness merit discussion. These include surveillance, the supply of drugs and vaccines, guidelines and manuals, training of human resources, and applied research.

How do international organizations decide where and when to intervene? The Ebola outbreak in Zaire attracted many groups. In contrast, two large epidemics of measles in Niger in 1991 and 1995 led to 100 000 cases, each with a probable case fatality rate of 10%, and yet very little was done, either at the national or the international level. We must find a way of ensuring that public health and epidemiological considerations determine whether or not an intervention is necessary and that such decisions are not driven mainly by research considerations, the media or politics.

The epidemic of meningitis in Nigeria in 1996 provides a good example of some of the problems of surveillance (WHO, 1996a). In Nigeria, an alert threshold of 15 cases per 100 000 per week during a period of two weeks was set as the threshold that would lead to vaccination at the district level. An evaluation performed by Epicentre and MSF in Kano State, Nigeria, showed that the peak of an epidemic in a district occurred a median of five weeks after the alert threshold had been crossed (AEDES, 1996). As a consequence of delays in decision-making and organisation, mass vaccination campaigns were started two to six weeks after the peak of the outbreak had been reached in 50% of the 28 local government areas (LGA) and only 37% of the target population was offered vaccination. The improper use of data for decision-making raises issues of training at national and international levels and probably also brings into question the feasibility of rapid mass immunization campaigns during meningitis epidemics. To be able to immunize a large population with less than one month's warning is a considerable challenge and requires excellent advance preparation.

Establishing a crisis committee with strong leadership, appropriate membership and a good plan of action is an essential component of epidemic management. It is important to identify in advance the potential partners who will be involved in making a response. This is not always done well and, despite the presence of representatives of major international organizations and NGOs in many countries, co-ordination is frequently initiated on the spot without careful preliminary preparation. The need for forward planning also applies to financial matters. This is illustrated by the way in which financial support was obtained by the various MSF sections during the Nigeria meningitis outbreak. Overall, 13 different donors provided 2.7 million ECUs of financial support to MSF and permitted almost four million vaccinations to be given in Nigeria. This was possible only because these contacts had been made in advance and because confidence between MSF and the donors had developed during past collaborations.

During the Nigeria outbreak of meningococcal meningitis, supply of vaccines and drugs was a major problem. Long-acting oily chloramphenicol was the recommended treatment; its story illustrates the perilous state of drugs whose market is mainly in the developing world. In 1992, MSF and Epicentre confirmed the efficacy of this drug in a clinical trial of 500 cases of meningitis seen in Niger and Mali. At the same time, the producer stopped the production of oily chloramphenicol. A lobby was then started by MSF and WHO which eventually led to resumption of production by two laboratories.

Ceftriaxone, the cost of which is rapidly decreasing, is an alternative drug, provided its production is not stopped also as it becomes used less widely in the industrialized world. These examples illustrate first the need for research on long-acting, cheap antibiotic treatments which are not supported at present, and secondly the necessity for international mechanisms to protect the emergence of orphan drugs which exist but are no longer produced.

Stockpiling is another important aspect of drug and vaccine supplies. WHO, in collaboration with various partners, has launched an action plan to secure 14 million doses of meningococcal vaccine for 1997 (WHO, 1997). In addition, taking the example of the Pan American Health Organization (PAHO) and several NGOs, stocks of essential drugs are being built up in targeted areas. These initiatives should probably be extended to other diseases. Finally, quality control requires a strong international commitment, for fake antibiotics and vaccines are now sold in many countries. We do not want to see again the appearance of the fake meningococcal vaccines that were used in Nigeria during the 1996 epidemic.

Health professionals like writing guidelines and manuals. Hundreds of guidelines have been created covering areas such as disease prevention and control, laboratory support, management and training. Many of these are, unfortunately, agency-specific and many agencies tend to reinvent guidelines, and to update and improve them. Some rationalization is needed. We need to be sure that manuals fit needs and that they are compatible with the other aspects of preparedness such as essential drug list, treatment protocols, and training.

Training is an important aspect of preparedness. Short courses proliferate like manuals. Many are very good; they ensure donor visibility and are popular among participants for many reasons. However, these short courses have limitations and we need to support the development of long-term practical field training programmes such as that of the epidemic intelligence service (EIS) in the US, the European programme for intervention epidemiology training (EPIET) and other worldwide field epidemiology training programmes (FETP), provided that these contribute to sustainable and appropriately financed public health programmes.

Collaboration is needed as much for research as for training. A lot of criticism was raised of the way the response to the cholera epidemic in Goma in July 1994 was handled. In particular, several researchers argued that those in the field should have used the new killed whole-cell B-subunit vaccine proposed by the US army. To help to solve this issue a cost-effectiveness study was done by MSF, Epicentre and the US National Institutes of Health (NIH) (Erikson, 1996). This compared the effectiveness and cost of four strategies: a presumptive treatment of cholera as soon as it was suspected (treatment centres established in advance), a reactive treatment after the start of the epidemic, a pre-emptive vaccination campaign and a reactive vaccination campaign. The results of this review suggested that the pre-emptive treatment strategy was the most cost-effective, supporting the activities of many NGOs in their preparedness strategies. This type of collaboration between NGOs and scientific institutions should definitely be developed to evaluate and improve operational programmes.

Role of NGOs

What role can NGOs play in co-ordination of the response to major international emergencies? Many NGOs have been created to fill a gap, to do what governments or large international institutions could not or did not want to do (MSF, 1996). NGOs are now well known for their mobility, flexibility and their logistical and training capacities. One of their major strengths is the ability of one NGO to cover the various components required for a successful response. In addition, major NGOs frequently base their decisions on whether or not to mount an intervention on a solid knowledge of the geopolitical issues. Finally, they have shown that they can play an important role in surveillance and early warning. NGOs are popular, maybe too much so. They should not be expected to replace or mask the lack of involvement by governments and major international institutions. The Great Lake crisis has illustrated clearly the limitations of NGOs acting alone without a strong international political mandate. There is definitely an important role for NGOs, which need to maintain their independence.

Role of WHO

Few dispute the need for a major United Nations agency in co-ordinating a response to a major epidemic (Toole, 1997). WHO has the mandate to take on this role, and the Kikwit experience has shown that experienced personnel from WHO can do this successfully (WHO, 1996b). However, the role of WHO in co-ordinating on-site responses to emergencies such as epidemics has, during the past two decades, been inconsistent and the organization has not gained the level of respect that it has achieved in other settings. With regards to preparedness, PAHO has probably been the most successful regional office, and its co-ordinating role is well respected among national governments. The effective co-ordination of responses to epidemics requires persons with very specific technical, managerial and interpersonal skills who can win the confidence of the various partners involved in response to epidemic threats. The recent creation of EMC is probably driving WHO in the right direction. However, to achieve efficient co-ordination successfully, WHO Geneva should probably strengthen its collaboration with regional and country-specific offices. In that respect the organizational structure of WHO sometimes limits its capacity to respond promptly and effectively, particularly with regard to its almost autonomous regional offices and its country offices, usually located within the Ministry of Health. Finally, there is still some room for improvement regarding the collaboration between UN agencies. For example, in order to avoid duplication of efforts, WHO, UNICEF and UNHCR could jointly develop an international roster of experienced and qualified specialists upon which each agency could draw during epidemics.

This paper has tried to describe and discuss some of the technical and organizational issues raised in co-ordination of the international responses to epidemics. However, the implementation of preventive measures still remains the best tool currently available. In addition, all partners involved should recognise that, whatever the quality of our technical response, it will be useless without strong political support.

References

AEDES. Meningitis epidemic in Nigeria, 1996. Evaluation of the MSF operation in North Nigeria from February to May 1996. Evaluation report, 1996

Erikson J. The international response to conflict and genocide: lessons from the Rwanda experience. Joint evaluation of emergency assistance to Rwanda. Synthesis Report, March 1996

Medecins sans Frontières (MSF). Operational responses to epidemics in developing countries. International symposium, Paris. MSF Report, 25 October 1996

Toole M. Health co-ordination in emergencies: options for the role of WHO. Concept paper. March 1997

World Health Organization (WHO). Report of the evaluation of the response to the cerebrospinal meningitis epidemic (CSM) in Nigeria, September 1996. Geneva: World Health Organization, 1996a

World Health Organization (WHO). *Ebola Viral Haemorrhagic Fever Epidemic, Kikwit (Bandundu) Zaire, 1995. Final Report*. Brazzaville: WHO Regional Office for Africa, 1996b
World Health Organization (WHO). International coordinating group on vaccine provision for meningitis control. Summary report, 16–17 January 1997

Discussion

Gilbert Mpigika

Malaria Control Unit, Ministry of Health, Entebbe, Uganda

In his paper, Dr Moren set out the essential components for a response to an outbreak or an epidemic. These include the existence of an effective disease surveillance and early warning system, a local public health laboratory able to investigate an outbreak—with help from an international laboratory when required—and the existence of a multisectoral national committee. The latter should be responsible for personnel, emergency funds, supplies, guidelines and communications with the media and the public.

In Uganda, a system has been established for dealing with epidemic and other important infectious diseases that involves the components of the health system and which meets many of the requirements set out by Dr Moren. At the central level, a National Task Force has been established which includes representatives of the Ministry of Health, other ministries, international organizations (WHO, UNICEF, USAID, UNHCR), NGOs (MSF, World Vision, Uganda Red Cross and others) and the Central Public Health Laboratory. The National Committee works closely with the district health team and hospital in the area of an outbreak. Finally, the community is fully represented in control by the inclusion of local leaders. The National Task Force has been active in the management of outbreaks of meningococcal meningitis, cholera and malaria and is involved in the guinea worm eradication programme.

Improvement of outbreak management and prevention in Uganda will require continuing political commitment of the Government, more training of health workers on the details of the epidemic control plan, improvement of disease surveillance at routine health facilities and education of the public on ways in which outbreaks can be detected and prevented.

13
Economic aspects of *E. coli* O157:H7: disease outcome trees, risk, uncertainty, and the social cost of disease estimates

Tanya Roberts, Jean Buzby, Jordan Lin, Peggy Nunnery*, Paul Mead[†] and Phillip I. Tarr[‡]

*The Economic Research Service, and *The Food Safety and Inspection Service, US Department of Agriculture, Washington DC, USA, [†]Centers for Disease Control and Prevention, Atlanta and [‡]University of Washington School of Medicine, Seattle, USA*

Economists have a variety of roles to play in public health. We bring a systems view to analysis of health care options, from prevention to treatment, in either the public or the private sector. Our cost and benefit estimates are useful in evaluating options, managing risks, and setting priorities. Economists depend for their analyses on data that the health system generates.

We illustrate seven critical issues in performing economic analyses for foodborne pathogens, using the emerging pathogen *Escherichia coli* O157:H7 as an example (Figure 13.1). This is an important example because outbreaks of *E. coli* O157:H7 disease have led to a reassessment of several aspects of food safety (Tenover and Hughes, 1996). *E. coli* O157:H7 can cause death in children and chronic kidney failure, making control of this pathogen a high priority in the USA (Besser *et al*, 1993; Bell *et al*, 1994; CDC, 1994; Tarr *et al*, 1997). Parents of some of these affected children have formed 'Safe Tables Our Priority' (STOP), a new type of lobbying group in the food safety arena (Heersink, 1996). Outbreaks of infection with this pathogen and other verotoxigenic *E. coli* have also occurred recently in Australia (Goldwater and Bettelheim, 1994), the UK (Wall *et al*, 1996; Pennington Group, 1997), and Japan (Watanabe *et al*, 1996).

New and Resurgent Infections: Prediction, Detection and Management of Tomorrow's Epidemics.
Edited by B. Greenwood and K. De Cock. Published 1998 John Wiley & Sons Ltd.

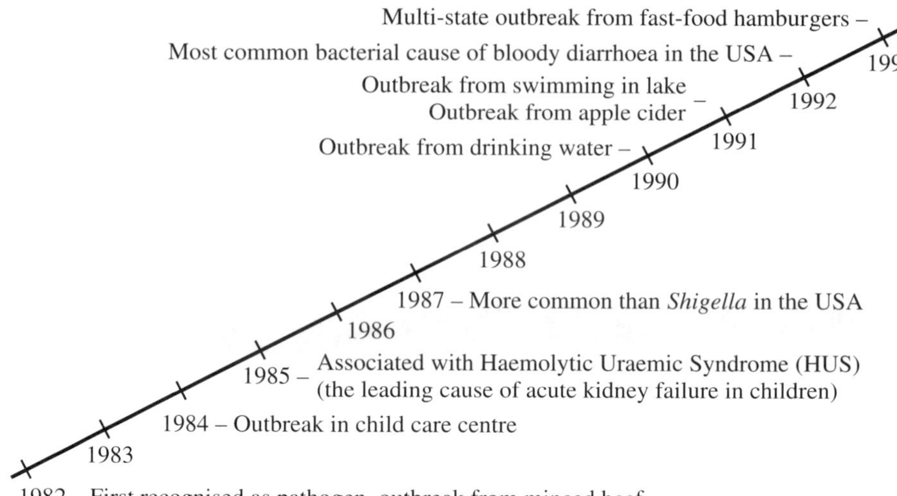

Figure 13.1 Emergence of *Escherichia coli* O157:H7
Source: CDC, 1994

How do we define foodborne disease? What data sources are available to estimate disease incidence and severity of outcome?

The broadest definition of foodborne disease includes:

- acute cases of diarrhoea and other illnesses that result from ingesting infected food. The US Council for Agricultural Science and Technology (CAST) identified 40 foodborne pathogens (1994);
- secondary cases that would not have happened if the initial case had not occurred. The classic example of this phenomenon is that of children in day care being infected by other children with *E. coli* O157:H7 disease. It is likely that many of these person-to-person cases originated with consumption of food contaminated with *E. coli* O157:H7;
- chronic sequelae, including autoimmune diseases, that have resulted from the foodborne infection
- workers who are exposed to the pathogen on the farm and during slaughter, transportation, and food preparation—these occupational exposures occur only because consumers are buying these foods.

The relative importance of each category of cases varies from pathogen to pathogen. While the greatest number of cases is usually the acute disease category, the greatest costs per case are associated with the occasional deaths and chronic complications. We believe that all these categories should be included in estimates of the annual incidence and cost of foodborne disease, wherever appropriate data is available.

Table 13.1. Advantages of data sets for acute foodborne illnesses

Data sources	Advantage	Cost
Outbreak data	Identifies common-source outbreaks that typically are large or serious enough to justify an investigation and identify some foodborne cases	Medium
Laboratory surveillance	Identifies foodborne pathogens causing moderate to severe symptoms and is useful for quantitative risk assessment	High
Review of medical cases in the literature	May discover new diseases, pathologies and severities, but is quite general	Low
Monitoring data from hospitals and public surveys	Identifies illnesses and deaths but often not specific foodborne pathogens	Medium
Sentinel county data and special epidemiological surveys	Identify case numbers, severity distributions, deaths, and may identify food vehicles. Useful for qualitative risk assessment	High

Source: CAST (1994)

In the USA, data on acute foodborne illnesses are derived from several different types of source (Table 13.1). Many data sources are designed primarily for purposes other than estimating national incidence, and may be inaccurate. For example, data on outbreaks, although useful for identifying trends in the sources of infection, do not provide data on the incidence of infection. Reliable estimates of population risks can only be derived from active surveillance systems. These systems tend to be labour-intensive and relatively costly. One example is the UK Department of Health survey of 200 000 people for intestinal infectious disease.

Another such system is the Foodborne Disease Active Surveillance Network (FoodNet), conducted by CDC with state health officials, with funding from CDC, the Food Safety and Inspection Service in the US Department of Agriculture and the Food and Drug Administration in the US Department of Health and Human Services (USDA: HHS: EPA, 1997). FoodNet employs active surveillance for foodborne diseases in a population of 13 million, together with epidemiological studies designed to help public health officials obtain a better understanding of the epidemiology of foodborne diseases in the USA. FoodNet provides a network for responding to new and emerging foodborne diseases of national importance and identifying the source of specific foodborne diseases. Because it is specifically designed to take measurements at multiple levels in the surveillance pyramid (Figure 13.2), FoodNet will provide much more detailed information on the overall burden of foodborne disease.

Based on preliminary results for 1996, the average risk to an individual living in a FoodNet site of becoming ill and having a positive stool culture for *E. coli* O157:H7 is 0.0029% per year (US Department of Health and Human Services, 1996). Extrapolating to the US population yields a rough national estimate of

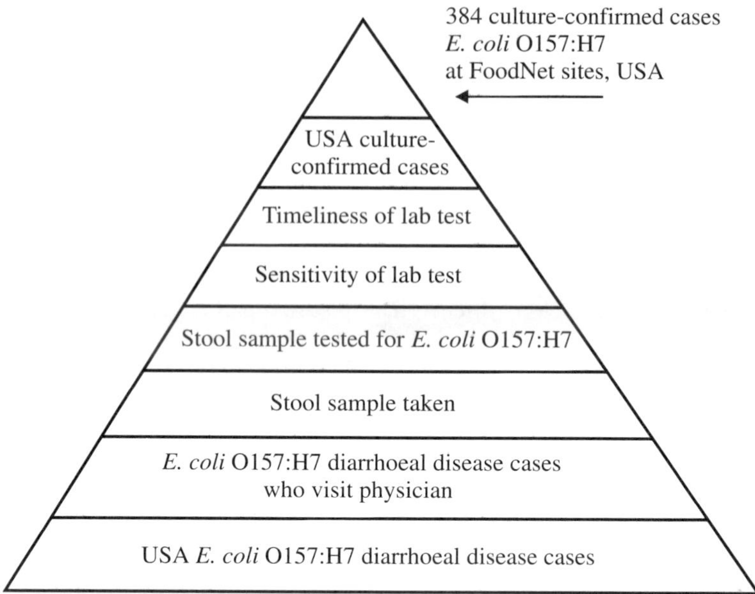

Figure 13.2 The surveillance pyramid

7540 culture-confirmed cases annually (Table 13.2). It is important to recognise that the number of culture-confirmed cases is known to be markedly smaller than the actual number of cases. Studies of *Salmonella* surveillance have shown that only one in 20 cases of infection is confirmed by culture (Chalker and Blaser, 1988).

It is also important to recognise that estimates of average risk hide considerable variability in risk between sites. Part of this variability may reflect the different case histories and surveillance capabilities for this disease. It is unlikely, however, that these account for all of the variability between sites. In a multi-centre study in which all stool specimens were routinely tested for *E. coli* O157:H7 the organism was isolated significantly more often from stool specimens collected in the northern states (Slutsker *et al*, 1997). To enhance further the generalizability of FoodNet data for the USA, President Clinton's 1997 Food Safety Initiative proposal (USDA:HHS:EPA, 1997) recommends expanding the FoodNet system from five to eight sites. Two additional sites have already been added—counties in New York and Maryland.

What epidemiological information is there on pathogen sources and levels, infectious dose, susceptibility of different demographic groups, etc?

Information about the source of *E. coli* O157:H7 infections is derived primarily from outbreak investigations. Most outbreaks of *E. coli* O157:H7 in the USA

Table 13.2 US Sentinel Site Surveillance, laboratory-confirmed cases for *E. coli* O157:H7, 1996

Site location	Population	Cases	Rate (%)	Cases extrapolated to the US*
Minnesota	4 375 099	238	0.0054	14 040
Oregon	2 842 321	75	0.0026	6 670
Connecticut	1 656 002	34	0.0021	5 460
California	2 003 141	22	0.0011	2 860
Georgia	2 344 514	15	0.0006	1 560
Total	13 221 077	384	0.0029	7 540

*Based on a US population of 260 million

have been linked to consumption of foods derived from cattle, such as lightly cooked minced beef or raw milk (USDA:APHIS:VS, 1994; Griffin and Tauxe, 1991). Meat, especially minced beef, has also been implicated as an important source of human infection (Le Saux *et al*, 1993; Mead *et al*, 1997). These findings are consistent with the knowledge that *E. coli* O157:H7 can live harmlessly in the gastrointestinal tracts of calves and other farm animals (Brown *et al*, 1997) and that cattle are an important reservoir for the organism (Hancock *et al*, 1994).

Other foods implicated as vehicles of infection in outbreaks and sporadic cases include apple cider, potatoes, dressing containing mayonnaise, pea salad, cantaloupe, unpasteurised apple juice, lettuce and venison (Griffin and Tauxe, 1991; Ackers *et al*, 1996; Keene *et al*, 1997). In most instances, these foods are known or believed to have been contaminated through contact with meat products or manure. Several outbreaks have been related to person-to-person transmission, especially in day-care settings (Griffin and Tauxe, 1991). Although less commonly implicated, contaminated water has also been documented as a source of both sporadic cases and outbreaks (Swerdlow *et al*, 1992; Keene *et al*, 1994).

Infectious dose is a complicated issue that makes it difficult to interpret the implications of various levels of contamination in food. CAST (1994) lists microbial, host, dietary and geographical factors which can influence the probability of foodborne infection or the severity of illness. The CAST report estimates that the infectious dose for *E. coli* O157:H7 illness is in the range of 10 to 1000 colony-forming units.

Modellers of foodborne diseases have to make several decisions about the structure of their models when dealing with infectious doses. These include:

- determining how to handle assumptions about the number of pathogens ingested: some models assume that there is no destruction of pathogen in the host's body; other models use epidemiological data to set a threshold to approximate an infectious dose; and in theory, the most elegant model would formally estimate the probability distribution that one or more pathogenic

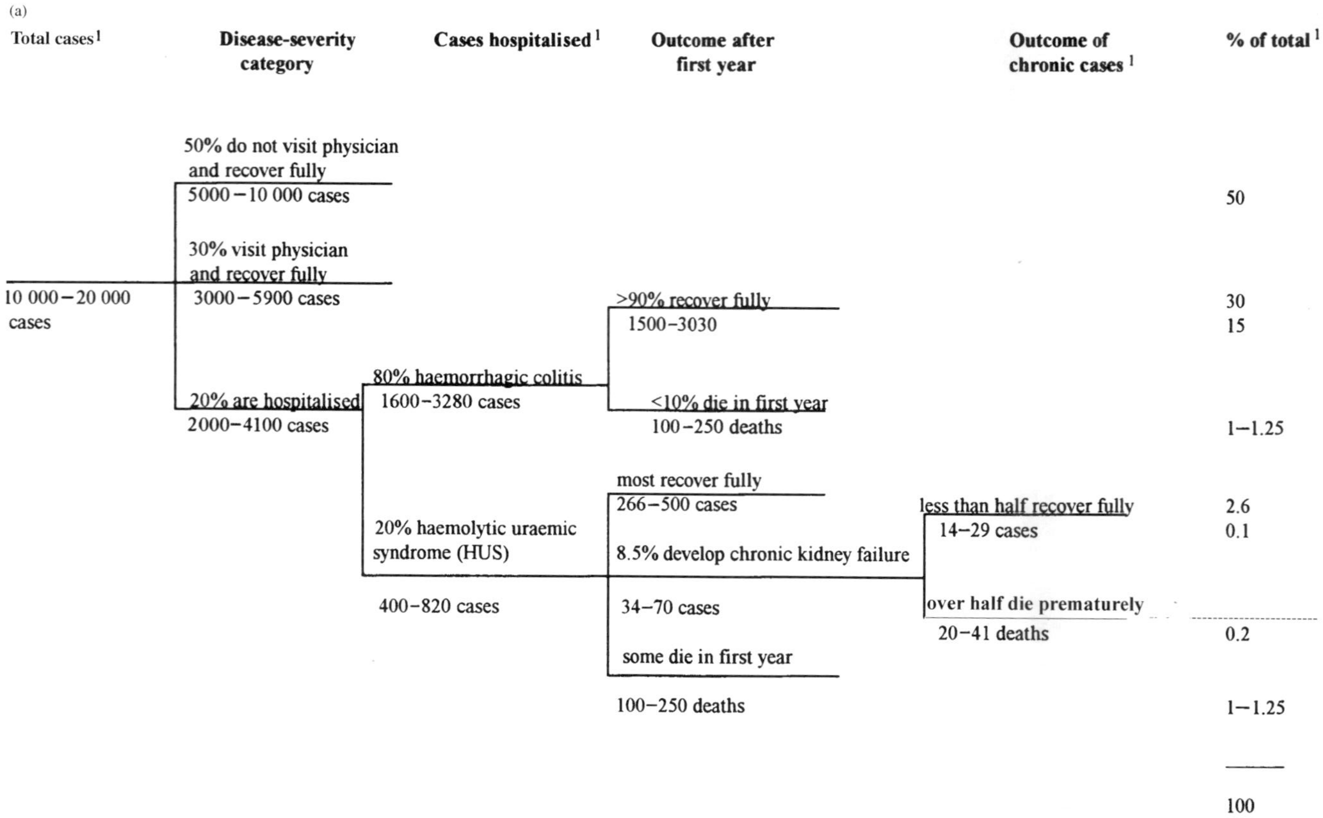

(a)

Total cases[1]	Disease-severity category	Cases hospitalised[1]	Outcome after first year	Outcome of chronic cases[1]	% of total[1]
	50% do not visit physician and recover fully 5000 − 10 000 cases				50
	30% visit physician and recover fully 3000 − 5900 cases				30
10 000 − 20 000 cases	20% are hospitalised 2000–4100 cases	80% haemorrhagic colitis 1600–3280 cases	>90% recover fully 1500–3030		15
			<10% die in first year 100–250 deaths		1–1.25
		20% haemolytic uraemic syndrome (HUS) 400–820 cases	most recover fully 266–500 cases		2.6
			8.5% develop chronic kidney failure 34–70 cases	less than half recover fully 14–29 cases	0.1
				over half die prematurely 20–41 deaths	0.2
			some die in first year 100–250 deaths		1–1.25
					100

Figure 13.3a Disease outcome tree for US *Escherichia coli* O157:H7 used in ERS cost-of-illness analysis, 1995.[1] Percentages and cases may be rounded

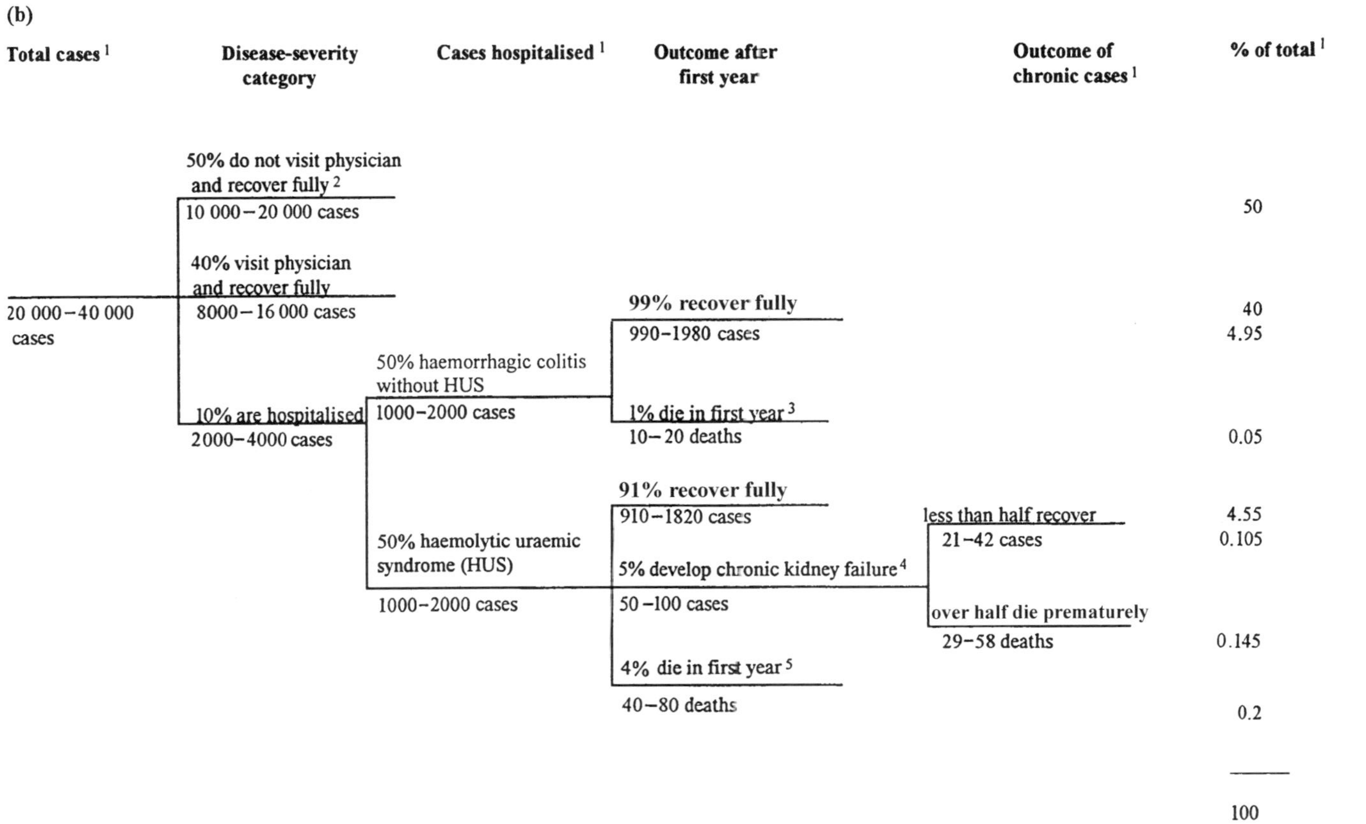

(b)

Total cases[1] | **Disease-severity category** | **Cases hospitalised**[1] | **Outcome after first year** | **Outcome of chronic cases**[1] | **% of total**[1]

20 000–40 000 cases

50% do not visit physician and recover fully[2]
10 000–20 000 cases — 50

40% visit physician and recover fully
8000–16 000 cases — 40

10% are hospitalised
2000–4000 cases

50% haemorrhagic colitis without HUS
1000–2000 cases

99% recover fully
990–1980 cases — 4.95

1% die in first year[3]
10–20 deaths — 0.05

50% haemolytic uraemic syndrome (HUS)
1000–2000 cases

91% recover fully
910–1820 cases — 4.55

5% develop chronic kidney failure[4]
50–100 cases

less than half recover
21–42 cases — 0.105

over half die prematurely
29–58 deaths — 0.145

4% die in first year[5]
40–80 deaths — 0.2

100

Figure 13.3b Suggested modifications to disease outcome tree for US *Escherechia coli* O157:H7, 1997. [1]Percentages and cases may be rounded; [2]Cieslak *et al.*, 1997; [3]Boyce *et al.*, 1995; Ryan *et al.*, 1986. Deaths also include possible undiagnosed deaths (HO *et al.*, 1988); [4]Or develop severe neurological impairments (Siegler *et al.*, 1994); [5]Siegler *et al.*, 1994; Martin *et al.*, 1990

organisms can find an appropriate spot in the body to attach and cause infection, toxicoinfection, or intoxication (See CAST (1994) for a discussion of the body defences against pathogens);
- decide whether infection, acute illness, chronic illness, or carrier status is the pathogen–host process being modelled. In infection, the host response may be so successful in fighting off the pathogen that disease does not occur, but an autoimmune response could be triggered that would result in chronic complications, such as arthritis or Guillain–Barré syndrome (Smith and Fratamico, in press);
- determine whether risks are being modelled for an average individual or a high-risk individual with some of the host characteristics listed by CAST (1994).

Another set of risk modelling issues deals with changes in the number of pathogens due to growth or destruction during food production, processing and preparation. From a public health perspective, quantitative risk assessment is hindered by lack of publicly available data and a shortage of complete models. These problems add to the uncertainties about infectious dose estimates. Efforts are being made to model changes in *E. coli* O157:H7 pathogen counts with the aid of predictive microbiology (e.g. GB ACMSF, 1995; Cassin *et al*, 1997; Marks *et al*, 1997).

How do we construct a disease outcome tree that includes all acute cases and associated chronic complications?

Figure 13.3a is the disease outcome tree for *E. coli* O157:H7 that the Economic Research Service (ERS) of the US Department of Agriculture used in its economic analysis (Buzby and Roberts, 1996, updated from Buzby *et al*, 1996). The disease outcome tree starts with the American Gastroenterological Association's (1995) estimate of 10 000–20 000 annual cases in the USA. These cases are divided into three severity groups: those who do not consult a physician, those who consult a physician and are treated as outpatients, and those who are admitted to a hospital. All those admitted to a hospital are assumed to have haemorraghic colitis, some of whom also develop haemolytic uraemic syndrome (HUS) or kidney failure. Some of the hospitalized cases die and some of the patients with HUS develop lifelong complications. We have found this disease outcome tree useful in organizing the medical data available and evaluating the completeness of these data. As we improve our databases and build better collaborations with the medical and epidemiological community, this disease outcome tree will be improved. In particular, we hope to expand the tree to include surveillance endpoints, in addition to the current clinical outcomes.

How might the disease outcome tree be revised and improved to incorporate the new data from FoodNet and the medical literature? Although the original tree began with an estimate of 10 000–20 000 cases in the general population, this

Table 13.3 Social costs of foodborne illness

Human illness costs:
Medical costs
Income or productivity loss for ill person or person dying, and caregiver for ill person
Other illness costs
Psychological costs
Averting behaviour costs (e.g. extra cleaning/cooking time costs)
Altruism (willingness to pay for others to avoid illness)
Industrial costs:
Impact of pathogens on animal production costs (e.g. costs of disposal of contaminated animals)
Control costs for pathogens at all links in the food chain (e.g. new processing procedures)
Outbreak costs (e.g. herd slaughter/product recall)
Regulatory and public health sector costs for foodborne pathogens
Disease surveillance costs
Research
Outbreak
Other considerations

estimate is actually based on patients who seek medical care (MacDonald *et al*, 1988). Thus, it would be more appropriate to use this estimate for the number of people seeking care, and to assume that the number of cases in the general population is higher still (see the possible revisions to the tree in Figure 13.3b). Cieslak (1997) and colleagues' investigation of an unnoticed outbreak of *E. coli* O157:H7 in Las Vegas revealed that 45% of ill persons had not sought medical care. Our extrapolation of 1996 FoodNet data suggests there may be 7540 culture-confirmed cases in the US annually. This number represents an underestimate of the true number of physician visits, however, as not all patients who visit a doctor for diarrhoea are cultured for *E. coli* O157:H7 (Figure 13.2).

While this first modification suggests that illness is more common than previously assumed, there is evidence that the death rate may be lower than originally stated, especially among patients with haemorrhagic colitis in the absence of HUS. Revised estimates are shown in Figure 13.3b, and yield a total death rate of 0.8% among patients seeking medical care. The new figures compare more favourably with recent FoodNet results. Of the 384 culture-confirmed *E. coli* O157:H7 illnesses identified through FoodNet, only two (0.5%) resulted in death in the first year. Assuming that there are 10 000–20 000 cases who seek medical care each year, this figure translates to 50–100 acute illness deaths in the USA annually. In addition, some undetermined number of cases which end in death may not receive medical care and/or may not be recognised as due to a foodborne pathogen (Ho *et al*, 1988).

Table 13.4 Estimated costs of selected foodborne pathogens in the US, 1995

Pathogen	Estimated foodborne illness		Estimated foodborne illness costs (billions of dollars)	
Disease/complication	Cases (*n*)	Deaths (*n*)	Assuming Landefeld & Seskin[a]	Assuming US $5 million/life[b]
Bacteria				
Campylobacter jejuni or *coli*				
Campylobacteriosis	1100 000–7000 000	110–511	0.7–4.3	1.2–6.6
Clostridium perfringens				
C. perfringens intoxications	10 000	100	0.1	0.5
Escherichia coli O157:H7				
E. coli O157:H7 disease	8000–16 000	80–200	0.1–0.3	0.4–1.0
Hemolytic uremic syndrome[c]	320–656	96–233	0.2–0.4	0.5–1.2
Subtotal	N/A	176–433	0.3–0.7	0.9–2.2
Listeria monocytogenes[d]				
Listeriosis	928–1767	230–485	0.12–0.25	1.2–2.2
Complications	22–41	0	0.03–0.05	0.1–0.2
Subtotal	N/A	230–485	0.1–0.3	1.3–2.4
Salmonella (non-typhoid)				
Salmonellosis	696 000–3840 000	870–1920	0.9–3.5	4.8–12.2
Staphylococcus aureus				
S. aureus intoxications	1513 000	454	1.2	3.3
Parasite				
Toxoplasma gondii[e]				
Toxoplasmosis	217	40	0.04	0.1
Complications	1541	0	3.15	7.6
Subtotal	1581	40	3.2	7.7
Total	3300 000–12 300 000	1900–3900	6.5–13.3	19.7–34.9

Cost estimates are in 1995 dollars. N/A means not applicable.
[a]Assuming Landefeld and Seskin (1992); this human capital approach, increased by a willingness to pay multiplier, estimates the value of a statistical life, depending on age, to range from roughly US $15 000 to US $1 979 000 in 1995 dollars.
[b]The US $5 million value of a statistical life used here was estimated from wage-risk studies.
[c]Kidney failure.
[d]Only includes hospitalized patients because of data limitations.
[e]Only includes toxoplasmosis cases related to foetuses and newborn children who may become blind or mentally retarded. Does not include all other cases of toxoplasmosis. Another high-risk group for this parasite is the immunocompromised, such as patients with AIDS. Some cases do not have noticeable acute

What economic valuation methods do we use to estimate the societal benefits of reducing *E. coli* O157:H7 and other foodborne pathogens?

Economic theory provides a precise framework to associate the benefits of risk reduction with the amount that people are willing to pay to achieve the reduction, and suggests methods of measuring those benefits (Just *et al*, 1982). As is often the case, some key theoretical constructs cannot be observed and, as a result, economists use practical applications of the theory to approximate the theoretically appropriate measure. The practical applications for human illnesses can be grouped into two primary methods of benefit estimation, the willingness-to-pay (WTP) method and the cost-of-illness (COI) method.

The WTP method aims to estimate the value that individuals place on reductions in risk. Recent attention in estimating WTP for reducing risks to life has focused on 'risk premiums' in labour markets. These studies derive the value of risk reduction by estimating statistically the effect of occupational mortality and injury risks on wages. Typically, employers must offer workers higher wages to induce them to take a job with some injury and mortality risks, as opposed to a similar job with no such risks. The 'risk premium' is then the increased wage needed to attract workers to riskier jobs (Buzby *et al*, 1996).

The COI method estimates society's resources expended on the human illness and these estimates can be used to generate the benefits of risk reduction. While in theory many categories of costs listed in Table 13.3 could be considered, in practice the COI method is generally limited to estimates of medical expenses and productivity losses (where work is missed because of illness). The advantage of this method over the WTP method lies in data reliability and availability. Some authors (e.g. Harrington and Portney, 1987) argue that COI can serve as a lower bound estimate for willingness to pay.

What are the estimates of the societal costs of *E. coli* O157:H7 and other foodborne pathogens?

ERS used the COI method to estimate the societal costs for seven foodborne pathogens in the USA—*Campylobacter jejuni, Clostridium perfringens, E. coli* O157:H7, *Listeria monocytogenes, Salmonella, Staphylococcus aureus* and *Toxoplasma gondii* (Buzby *et al*, 1996; Buzby and Roberts 1996). In general, for each foodborne illness, cases were divided into five severity groups: those who did not visit a physician, those who visited a physician, those who were hospitalized, those who died prematurely because of their illness, and those who developed chronic complications. For each severity group, medical costs were estimated for physician and hospital services, supplies, medications, and special procedures unique to treating that particular foodborne illness. Such costs reflect the number of days of a medical service/treatment, the average cost per service/treatment, and the number of patients receiving such service/treatment.

Table 13.5 Cost summary for US *E. coli* O157:H7 disease cases, 1995

		Estimated illness costs (millions of dollars)[a]	
Cost category	Estimated cases (*n*)	Assuming Landefeld and Seskin	Asssuming US $5 million/life
Medical costs[b]			
Acute illness medical costs			
No physician visit	5000–10 000	0.0	0.0
Physician visit	3000–5900	0.5–1.9	0.5–1.9
Hospitalized—haemorrhagic colitis	1600–3280	20.2–41.4	20.2–41.4
Hospitalized—HUS	400–820	15.8–32.5	15.8–32.5
Subtotal	10 000–20 000	36.5–75.8	36.5–75.8
Chronic illness medical costs			
Chronic cases (present value)	34–70	11.9–23.0	11.9–23.0
Total medical costs	N/A	48.4–98.8	48.4–98.8
Productivity losses[c]			
Acute illness productivity losses			
No physician visit	5000–10 000	1.2–2.4	1.2–2.4
Visited physician	3000–5900	1.5–2.9	1.5–2.9
Hospitalized—haemorrhagic colitis[d]	1500–3030	2.5–5.1	2.5–5.1
Hospitalized—HUS[d]	300–570	1.2–2.2	1.2–2.2
Deaths (present value)[d]	200–500	301.9–754.8	1000.0–2500.0
Subtotal	10 000–20 000	308.3–767.4	1006.4–2512.6
Chronic illness productivity losses			
Survivors (present value)	14–29	3.4–7.2	3.4–7.2
Deaths (present value)	20–41	20.4–39.1	63.5–122.8
Subtotal	34–70	23.8–46.3	66.9–129.9
Total productivity losses	N/A	332.1–813.7	1073.3–2642.5
Total	10 000–20 000	380.5–912.5	1121.7–2741.3
Assuming 80% are foodborne, foodborne costs (US$ billion) are:		0.3–0.7	0.9–2.2

Numbers may not total due to rounding. N/A = not applicable

[a] See footnote to Table 13.4

[b] Medical costs were estimated using data from the American Hospital Association's Hospital Statistics and the US Health Care Financing Administration

[c] Productivity losses were estimated using data from the US Bureau of Labor Statistics and Landefeld and Seskin's (1982) estimated values of statistical life. The 220–541 premature deaths include 200–500 deaths from the acute illness and 20–41 deaths from chronic complications.

[d] For the productivity loss section, hospitalized cases were divided into three categories: (1) hospitalized with haemorrhagic colitis and survived, (2) hospitalized with HUS and survived, and (3) hospitalized and died (i.e. deaths)

Most people with a foodborne illness miss only a few days of work and their productivity losses are represented by foregone daily wages estimated using US Bureau of Labor Statistics data. However, some patients die and some develop complications so that they either never return to work, regain only a portion of their pre-illness productivity, or switch to less demanding and lower paying jobs. The total cost of lost productivity is the sum for all individuals affected, including the patients and, in the case of ill children, their parents or paid caretakers.

For those who die or are unable to return to work because of their illness, ERS's COI analyses used two types of approaches as a proxy for these productivity losses. The first approach uses Landefeld and Seskin's (1982) estimates which represent an individual's lifetime stream of income (present value) if the illness had not occurred. These estimates depend on age and range from $15 000 to $1 979 000 per person (after updating to 1995 dollars). Using this first method, total annual costs of the seven foodborne illnesses in the USA ranged between US $6.5 and US $13.3 billion (Table 13.4).

The second ERS approach uses the 'risk premium' that is required to attract workers to risky jobs. Viscusi (1993) has reviewed the studies in the literature, and concluded that the results are reasonably consistent and indicate a labour market value of US $5 million per statistical life lost. This risk premium is essentially a WTP estimate so it incorporates other costs in addition to lost productivity. Using this second method, total annual costs increased to US $19.7–34.9 billion.

Both sets of estimates undervalue the true costs of all foodborne illnesses to society, however, because the analyses covered only seven pathogens—there are over 40 different foodborne pathogens believed to cause human illnesses (CAST, 1994). Estimated costs of illness would also increase if the costs for all complications linked to foodborne illnesses, such as arthritis, meningitis or Guillain–Barré syndrome were included. Estimated costs would also increase if more categories of social costs were estimated (Table 13.3).

Table 13.5 provides a detailed breakdown of the total annual US costs of *E. coli* O157:H7 disease from all sources (e.g. food, water, person-to-person) and estimated using the outcome tree illustrated in Figure 13.3a. Using the Landefeld and Seskin estimates in the COI analyses, total annual US costs were estimated at US $0.4–0.9 billion (1995 US$). Assuming 80% of the estimated human illnesses due to *E. coli* O157:H7 are attributed to food, the foodborne costs for *E. coli* O157:H7 are estimated at US $0.3–0.7 billion annually. Using the US $5 million estimate in the COI analyses, the high estimated costs for *E. coli* O157:H7 disease in the US estimates is US $1.1–2.7 billion annually (1995 US$), with an estimated US $0.9–2.2 billion attributed to food sources. The variability in cost estimates is about two-fold within methods (caused by differences in estimated incidence of disease) and three-fold between economic methods.

The assumption that 80% of all *E. coli* O157:H7 cases are from food (CDC, unpublished outbreak data) appears reasonable in light of the relatively low number of cases resulting from contaminated water and the estimate by Martin and colleagues (1990) that an upper bound of 16% of cases are from person-to-person transmission in day-care centres. This estimate also omits the extra costs of testing for other foodborne pathogens in an outbreak setting that Del Beccaro *et al.* (1995) quantified for the 1993 Seattle outbreak. Another cost category excluded is the settlement of legal liability cases; for example, the City of Sakai, Japan, authorised payment of 810 000 000 yen (equivalent to US $6 500 000) on the following payment schedule: 21 000 yen/day to those hospitalized with HUS, 16 000 yen/day to those hospitalized without HUS, 8 000 yen/day to outpatients; compensation for death and chronic complications is determined on a case-by-case basis (Dr Takuji Sakurai, personal communication).

How do we anticipate emerging foodborne pathogens and deal with uncertainty and variability in our analyses?

There are several sources of uncertainty in our attempts to analyse risks from foodborne pathogens. The most difficult to anticipate is the emerging pathogen. Recent emerging pathogens include *E. coli* O157:H7, *Listeria monocytogenes*, *Campylobacter* species (MacDonald and Osterholm, 1993), *Toxoplasma gondii*, and *Salmonella enteritidis*. Enterococci are becoming 'increasingly resistant to multiple antimicrobial agents' (Tenover and Hughes, 1996) and this suggests the possibility that some enteric foodborne pathogens might become increasingly resistant to antibiotics and limit human treatment options. Also of concern are the as yet unidentified agents that cause bovine spongiform encephalitis (BSE) and Brainerd diarrhoea, which are plausibly transmissible to the human population via food.

Increased investment in surveillance databases from farm to table, literature reviews on chronic complications and their possible links to foodborne pathogens, and risk assessment models are likely to decrease the probability of being surprised by new pathogens and increase our ability to design and evaluate cost-beneficial interventions. Multidisciplinary input is required to develop databases and construct models (Roberts *et al*, 1995). When we have enough data to build models or estimate human illness costs, some of the uncertainty (the unknown) can be defined mathematically as variability of parameters in the models (USPCCRARM, 1997). This variability can be captured in sensitivity analyses that use different values for major parameters in the models. For example, in the cost estimation we used two techniques for valuing a statistical life.

How can economics be useful in analysing food safety issues and in helping to determine food safety priorities?

Ideally, to understand better the true societal costs of foodborne illness in the US, costs should be estimated for all 40 or more known foodborne pathogens and their associated complications (CAST, 1994). Detailed economic estimates can clarify the consequences of infection. For example, foodborne congenital toxoplasmosis may appear to be of minor concern since the cases are few compared to salmonellosis and campylobacteriosis, but the high percentage of severe complications means that congenital toxoplasmosis is the most costly pathogen in Table 13.4. Another advantage of economic cost estimates is that all the cases ranging from mild to deadly, are captured in one estimate for each foodborne pathogen. These COI estimates can be used to estimate the benefits of a public health protection effort which can later be compared with the costs of implementing that effort.

Decision-makers have other considerations that also guide their priority lists for risk management, such as:

- concern about particular demographic groups,
- the level of safety that society prefers,
- societal preferences for public programmes versus private efforts to reach target levels of safety
- information about the trade-offs (cost, risk reduction) for different policy options.

Economic analysis of the costs of alternative policy options and their likely impact on the level of safety may influence both the target level of safety and the mix of public and private efforts chosen.

Discussion

New and re-emerging infections raise complex issues for those attempting to carry out economic evaluations and to design systems to improve public health. One of the primary issues is the lack of data on disease risks and severity, especially for emerging infections. In this paper, we presented a framework for economic evaluation of the societal costs of an emerging foodborne pathogen, *E. coli* O157:H7. In preparation for the economic analysis, we developed a disease outcome tree and used the best available epidemiological data on cases and severity outcomes (and we also suggested how the tree might be modified to incorporate new FoodNet and medical data). We discussed alternative economic methodologies for valuing risk reduction for foodborne disease, which result in a range of estimated costs of US $6.5 billion to US $35 billion annually for seven pathogens. The cost estimates based on risk premiums (a willingness-to-pay measure) have a more solid foundation in economic theory than those estimates which used the lifetime stream of income.

Knowledge of foodborne risks can be improved, at a cost, by expanding surveillance for human illness caused by foodborne pathogens and by expanding the monitoring of food to identify which foods are the vehicles for which pathogens (MacDonald and Osterholm, 1993). Case-control studies all along the food chain may identify which food production, consumption and food-handling procedures contribute to foodborne illness for specific pathogens (USDA:HHS:EPA,

1997). FoodNet is expected to provide valuable information about US practices regarding the handling and preparation of food.

Four goals identified by the World Health Organization (LeDuc, 1996) to combat emerging infectious diseases are to: 'strengthen global surveillance of infectious diseases; rebuild the international infrastructure necessary to recognize, report, and respond to emerging and resurgent infectious diseases; foster applied research and enhance the international capacity for infectious disease prevention and control.' To this list of goals, we add the development of risk modelling to identify control options. In addition, it is important to consider economic analysis of public and private control options to determine which are the most cost-beneficial. Recent US actions include Hazard Analysis and Critical Control Point (HACCP) regulations for seafood and for meat and poultry. The President's Food Safety Initiative, if implemented, will increase US resources devoted to improving food safety.

Note

The views expressed are those of the authors and do not represent the views of their employers. We also appreciated insightful review comments from Phyllis Sparling, FSIS/CDC, Dr Takuji Sakurai, Osaka, Japan, and Katherine Ralston and Ann Vandeman, ERS.

References

Ackers M, Mahon B, Leahy E *et al.* An outbreak of *Escherichia coli* O157:H7 infections associated with leaf lettuce consumption, western Montana. *Abstracts of the 36th Interscience Conference on Antimicrobial Agents and Chemotherapy, September 15–18 1996, New Orleans, Louisiana.* Washington, DC: American Society for Microbiology, 1996

American Gastroenterological Association (AGA). Consensus conference statement: *Escherichia coli* O157:H7 infections—an emerging national health crisis, July 11–13, 1994. *Gastroenterology*, 1995; **108:** 1923–1934

Bell BP, Goldoft M, Griffin PM *et al.* A multistate outbreak of *Escherichia coli* O157:H7—associated bloody diarrhea and hemolytic uremic syndrome from hamburgers. The Washington experience. *Journal of the American Medical Association*, 1994; **17**: 1349–1353

Besser RE, Lett SM, Weber JT *et al.* An outbreak of diarrhea and hemolytic uremic syndrome from *Escherichia coli* O157:H7 in fresh-pressed apple cider. *Journal of the American Medical Association*, 1993; **269**: 2217–2220

Boyce TG, Swerdlow DL, Griffin PM, *Escherichia coli* O157: H7 and the hemolytic- uremic syndrome. *New England Journal of Medicine*, 1995; **333**: 364–368.

Brown CA, Harmon BG, Zhao T, Doyle MP. Experimental *Escherichia coli* O157:H7 carriage in calves. *Applied and Environmental Microbiology*, 1997; **63:** 27–32

Buzby JC, Roberts T. ERS updates U.S. foodborne disease costs for seven pathogens. *FoodReview*, Washington DC: US Department of Agriculture, Economic Research Service, Sept–Dec 1996; **19**: 20–25

Buzby JC, Roberts T, Lin JC-T, MacDonald JM. *Bacterial foodborne disease: medical costs and productivity losses.* Washington, DC: US Department of Agriculture, Economic Research Service, AER No. 741, August 1996

Cassin MH, Lammerding AM, Todd ECD, Ross W, McColl RS. Quantitative risk assessment of *E. coli* O157:H7 in ground beef hamburgers. Health Canada, 1997, unpublished paper

CAST Report. *Foodborne pathogens: risks and consequences.* Task Force Report No. 122, Ames, Iowa, USA: Council for Agricultural Science and Technology, Sept 1994

Centers for Disease Control and Prevention (CDC). *Addressing emerging infectious disease threats: a prevention strategy for the United States.* Atlanta, GA: US Department of Health and Human Services, Public Health Service, 1994, p.11

Chalker RB, Blaser MJ. A review of human salmonellosis: III. Magnitude of *Salmonella* infection in the United States. *Reviews of Infectious Diseases*, 1988; **10**: 111–124

Cieslak PR, Noble SJ, Maxson DJ et al. Hamburger-associated *Escherichia coli* O157:H7 infection in Las Vegas: a hidden epidemic. *American Journal of Public Health*, 1997; 87: 176–180

Del Beccaro MA, Brownstein DR, Cummings P, Goldoft MJ, Quan L. Outbreak of *Escherichia coli* O157:H7 hemorrhagic colitis and hemolytic uremic syndrome: effect on use of a pediatric emergency department. *Annals of Emergency Medicine*, 1995; **26**:598–603

Goldwater PN, Bettelheim KA. The role of enterohaemorrhagic *E. coli* serotypes other than O157:H7 as causes of disease. In: Karmali MA, Goglio AG (eds), *Recent Advances in Verocytotoxin-producing* Escherichia coli *Infections.* 1994, pp 57–60

Great Britain Advisory Committee on the Microbial Safety of Food (GBACMSF). *Report on verocytotoxin-producing* Escherichia coli. London: HMSO, 1995

Griffin PM, Tauxe RV. The epidemiology of infections caused by *Escherichia coli* O157:H7, other enterohemorrhagic *E. coli*, and the associated hemolytic uremic syndrome. *Epidemiologic Reviews*, 1991; **13:** 60–98

Hancock DD, Besser TE, Kinsel ML. The prevalence of *Escherichia coli* O157:H7 in dairy and beef cattle in Washington State. *Epidemiology and Infection*, 1994; **113**: 199–207

Harrington W, Portney PR. Valuing the benefits of health and safety regulations. *Journal of Urban Economics*, 1987; **22:** 101–112

Heersink M. *E. coli* O157:H7: *The True Story of a Mothers Battle with a Killer Microbe.* Far Hills, NJ: New Horizon Press, 1996

Ho MS, Glass RI, Pinsky PF *et al.* Diarrheal deaths in American children. Are they preventable? *Journal of the American Medical Association*, 1988; **260**: 3281–3285

Just RE, Hueth DL, Schmitz A. *Applied Welfare Economics and Public Policy.* Englewood Cliffs, NJ: Prentice-Hall, 1982

Keene WE, McAnulty JM, Hoesly FC *et al.* A Swimming-associated outbreak of hemorragic colitis caused by *Escherichia coli* O157:H7 and *Shigella sonnei. New England Journal of Medicine* 1994; **331**. 579–584

Keene WE, Sazie E, Kok J *et al.* An outbreak of *Escherichia coli* O157:H7 infections traced to jerky made from deer meat. *Journal of the American Medical Association*, 1997; **277**: 1229–1231

Landefeld JS, Seskin EP. The economic value of life: linking theory to practice. *American Journal of Public Health*, 1982; **6**: 555–566

LeDuc JW. World Health Organization strategy for emerging infectious diseases. *Journal of the American Medical Association*, 1996; **275**: 318–320

Le Saux N, Spika JS, Friesen B *et al.* Ground beef consumption in noncommercial settings is a risk factor for sporadic *Escherichia coli* O157:H7 infection in Canada. *Journal of Infectious Diseases*, 1993; **167**: 500–502

MacDonald KL, O'Leary MJ, Cohen ML *et al. Escherichia coli* O157:H7, an emerging gastrointestinal pathogen. Results of a one-year, prospective, population-based study. *Journal of the American Medical Association*, 1988; **259**: 3567–3570

MacDonald KL, Osterholm MT. The emergence of *Escherichia coli* O157:H7 infection in the United States: the changing epidemiology of foodborne disease. *Journal of the American Medical Association*, 1993; **269:** 2264–2266

Marks HM, Coleman ME, Lin C-TJ, Roberts T. Topics in microbial risk assessment: dynamic flow tree modeling. *Risk Analysis*, 1997, in press

Martin DL, MacDonald KL, White KE, Soler JT, Osterholm MT. The epidemiology and clinical aspects of the hemolytic uremic syndrome in Minnesota. *New England Journal of Medicine*, 1990; **323:** 1161–1167

Mead PS, Finelli L, Lambert-Fair MA *et al.* Risk factors for sporadic infection with *Escherichia coli* O157:H7. *Archives of Internal Medicine*, 1997; **157**: 204–208

Pennington Group. *The Pennington Group: Report on the Circumstances Leading to the 1996 Outbreak of Infection with* E. coli *O157 in Central Scotland, the Implications for Food Safety and the Lessons to be Learned.* Edinburgh: The Stationery Office, 1997

Roberts T, Jensen H, Unnevehr L. (eds). *Tracking Foodborne Pathogens from Farm to Table: Data Needs to Evaluate Control Options.* Washington, DC: US Department of Agriculture, Economic Research Service Miscellaneous publication No 1532, Dec 1995

Ryan CA, Tauxe RV, Hosek GW *et al. Escherichia coli* O157:H7 diarrhea in a nursing home: clinical edpidemiological and pathological findings. *Journal of Infectious Diseases*, 1986; **154**: 631–638

Siegler RL, Pavia AT, Christofferson RD, Milligan MK. A 20-year population-based study of postdiarrheal hemolytic uremic syndrome in Utah. *Pediatrics*, 1994; **94**: 35–40

Slutsker L, Ries AA, Greene KD, Wells JG, Hutwagner L, Griffin PM. *Escherichia coli* O157:H7 diarrhea in the United States: clinical and epidemiological features. *Annals of Internal Medicine*, 1997: **126**: 505–513

Smith JL, Fratamico PM. Long-term consequences of foodborne disease. In: Lund B, Baird-Parker AC, Gould GW (eds). *Microbiology of Food.* London Chapman and Hall, in press

Swerdlow DL, Woodruff BA, Brady RC *et al.* A waterborne outbreak in Missouri of *Escherichia coli* O157:H7 associated with bloody diarrhea and death. *Annals of Internal Medicine*, 1992; **117:** 812–819

Tarr PI, Besser TE, Hancock DD, Keene WE, Goldoft M. Verotoxigenic *Escherichia coli* infection: United States overview. *Journal of Food Protection*, 1997, in press

Tenover FC, Hughes JM. The challenges of emerging infectious diseases. Development and spread of multiply-resistant bacterial pathogens. *Journal of the American Medical Association*, 1996; **275:** 300–304

USDA:APHIS:VS. Escherichia coli *O157:H7: issues and ramifications.* Fort Collins, CO: US Department of Agriculture and US Animal and Plant Health Inspection Service, Centers for Epidemiology and Animal Health, March 1994

USDA:HHS:EPA. *U.S. Dept. of Agriculture, US Department of Health and Human Services, U.S. Environmental Protection Agency. Discussion draft and current thinking: a national food safety initiative.* 4 March, 1997

US Department of Health and Human Services. *Surveillance for outbreaks of* Escherichia coli *O157:H7 infection—preliminary summary of 1995 data.* Centers for Disease Control and Prevention (CDC), US Department of Health and Human Services. Correspondence from the CDC to state and territorial epidemiologists and public health laboratory directors, 21 March, 1996

US Presidential/Congressional Commission on Risk Assessment and Risk Management (USPCCRARM). Risk assessment and risk management in regulatory decision-making. Volume 2. Washington, DC, 1997

Viscusi WK. The value of risks to life and health. *Journal of Economic Literature*, 1993; **31:** 1912–1946

Wall PG, McDonnell RJ, Adak GK *et al.* General outbreaks of Vero cytotoxin producing *Escherichia coli* O157 in England and Wales from 1992 to 1994. *Communicable Disease Review*, 1996; **6**: R26–33

Watanabe H, Wada A, Inagaki Y, Itoh K, Tamura K. Outbreaks of enterohaemorrhagic *Escherichia coli* 0157:H7 by two different genotype strains in Japan, 1996. *Lancet*, 1996: **348**; 831–832

14
Reducing uncertainty in infectious disease control—the role of health economics research

Susan Foster

Department of Public Health and Policy, London School of Hygiene & Tropical Medicine, UK

Health economics has much to offer the field of infectious disease control, especially when questions of allocation of resources are involved. Although its roots go back to the 17th century, health economics is a relatively young discipline and most of the important work on the economics of infectious diseases has been done in the past 15–20 years—much of it supported by the UK Department for International Development (formerly the Overseas Development Administration), the WHO Special Programme for Research and Training in Tropical Diseases (TDR) or the World Bank. One of the main goals of economics is to provide information on which to base decisions about the allocation of scarce resources—frequently money, but also time, human resources, and other factors. When properly applied, health economics research can reduce uncertainty and reduce the risk of resources being used sub-optimally.

Three questions of interest to a health economist can be asked about a particular infectious disease.

1. Is its control a priority? For example, should more resources be devoted to control of malaria or to HIV/AIDS?
2. What approach or control strategy is most appropriate? For example, should this include a vertical or an integrated approach, and passive or active case finding?
3. Within each strategy, what are the options available at each step of the control procedure? What do they cost, and how can we choose between them?

New and Resurgent Infections: Prediction, Detection and Management of Tomorrow's Epidemics.
Edited by B. Greenwood and K. De Cock.

Table 14.1 The problems of achieving successful control of an infection such as tuberculosis (the Piot model)

- % for whom prevention fails
- % who are infected
- % aware of their infection (symptomatic)
- % who seek care for their infection/symptom
- % who get appropriate diagnosis of their infection
- % who get appropriate treatment for their infection
- % who comply with their treatment
- (% who tell partners or others at risk of the infection to get treatment)

Work on the global burden of disease which was done in preparation for the 1993 World Development Report addresses primarily the first question (World Bank, 1993). This chapter deals with the second two concerns—strategy and micro-level options.

The structure of this chapter draws upon the 'Piot model', which was originally proposed in the 1970s at WHO by Maurice Piot to illustrate the problems of tuberculosis control, and more recently applied to other diseases such as sexually transmitted diseases (STDs). Piot observed that a number of steps were involved in achieving successful control of an infectious disease. Many people with the disease (in this case TB) did not receive treatment, including some who came to the health services in search of a cure for their cough. There were many reasons for this, as things could go wrong at each step in the sequence. Table 14.1 provides a simplified version of Piot's basic model.

The potential problem areas for disease control vary from disease to disease. Thus, in the case of STDs a major problem is awareness of symptoms. In the cases of malaria, TB and STDs, diagnosis is a weak point. In the case of TB perhaps the weakest point is compliance or adherence with even 'short course' treatment.

The following are examples in which health economics research has made a contribution to reducing uncertainty at one or more levels in Piot's model.

Prevention

An example of secondary prevention—preventing people with an infection from becoming ill—is preventive therapy for tuberculosis in subjects with HIV infection. Not only does infection with HIV increase the risk of developing TB, but TB increases the rate of progression of HIV disease. The interaction of these two infections is bad for the patient and also bad for the community. It has been shown that under certain circumstances—for example in a situation in which there is a high risk that a person with HIV will infect a number of other people because of the nature of their work or their living circumstances—the benefits of isoniazid preventive therapy exceed its costs by a factor of as much as four. This takes account of the relatively low uptake of preventive therapy and low compliance, and of the need to test many in order to find a few eligible persons (Foster *et al*, 1997). People who are candidates for preventive therapy include teachers and students, health care workers, bus conductors, prisoners, soldiers, policemen and miners.

Screening for syphilis in pregnancy provides another example of the role of health economics in guiding policy on infectious disease prevention. The costs of screening for syphilis are relatively high in comparison to the costs of treatment, especially when the scarcity of laboratory technicians is taken into account. In areas with a prevalence of syphilis of the order of 10%, the economic case for presumptive treatment of *all* antenatal attenders is strong, especially when testing and treatment cannot be done during the same visit. Many women with a positive result fail to return for treatment, thus not only remaining untreated but also 'wasting' the cost of the testing. A major problem area is what to do about the untreated partners. An attempt to treat as many partners as possible must be set against the opportunity of treating nearly all mothers and babies.

Care-seeking behaviour

Many patients attempt self-treatment. Others ignore their symptoms until either the problem resolves or their symptoms become so serious that some kind of intervention is necessary. A major cause of delay in seeking care is its economic cost, both in terms of financial cost and in terms of lost time and its consequences for productivity. Other factors involved include distance from the nearest health services, the stigma of being diagnosed as a case of a particular infection, and poor attitude of health care staff. More attention is now being paid to these aspects of health care. Saunderson (1995) found in Uganda that expenditures by patients in seeking care for their TB accounted for over 70% of the total cost of treating the illness. Similarly, Needham *et al*, working in Lusaka, Zambia found that patients spent the equivalent of one and a half month's wages on seeking care prior to diagnosis; 38% of patients who delayed seeking treatment did so for financial reasons (Needham *et al*, submitted). This sample was drawn from people who were being seen at the chest clinic—what of the others who made similar expenditures but are yet to be diagnosed? It is unfortunate that so many patients spend so much of their household resources in obtaining a diagnosis and yet leave the health services without treatment.

Diagnosis

How much should be spent on improved diagnostics? How much is it worth improving microscopic diagnosis of TB and malaria? What is the role of new techniques such as the polymerase chain reaction (PCR)? Brinkmann and Brinkmann (1991) pointed out that, in Africa, when passive case detection is used, only 40–50% of cases of fever are caused by malaria and that in the dry season this figure may be as low as 30%. Using active case detection only 5% of patients

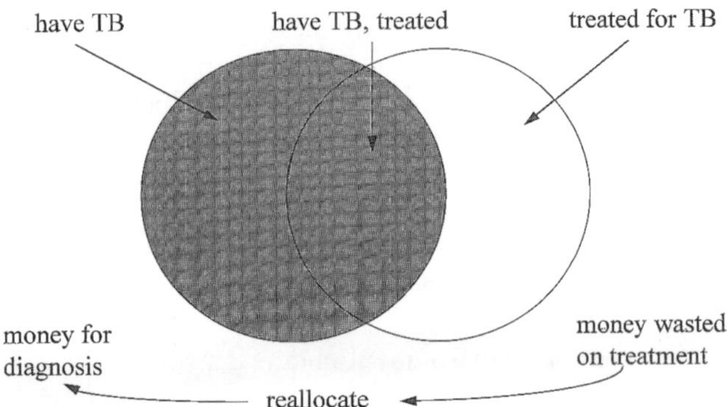

Figure 14.1 Use of resources in the control of tuberculosis

with fever had malaria and up to 95% of the drugs used for the treatment of malaria were wasted (Najera *et al*, 1992). In these circumstances the drug costs per case of *true* malaria were 20 times higher than the cost of a course of drugs. The more expensive the drug used, the greater the gains from more accurate diagnosis. An approach that was economically reasonable when chloroquine was the first-line drug may no longer be good practice.

The same problem applies in the case of tuberculosis. How many cases of TB are missed because the microscopist has had a long day or was just unlucky in examination of the specimen, and how many people who do not have TB are put on a 'short' six-month course of therapy, with all the attendant consequences for their family finances, their job, and their social circumstance? This is illustrated in Figure 14.1. The cost of treatment for TB can be substantial, including not only the costs of the drugs but also the cost of the health care, which may include hospitalization, needed for about 25–30% of very ill patients, and the costs to the patient and family, which may include the loss of a job or of a livelihood. In such cases better diagnosis is worth paying for.

In many cases a search for improved diagnostics is clearly needed but how much additional expenditure is economically justified, and how can this be calculated? To answer this question, Phillips and Phillips-Howard (1996) have proposed a simple rule. It is worth paying up to the cost of treatment minus the percentage of true cases divided by 100 ($Ct\ (100 - p)/100$) per diagnosis. For example, in an area where mefloquine is needed to treat malaria, (Ct = US$2.40) and 30% of suspected cases are confirmed, it would be worth paying up to US$1.68 per diagnosis for a sensitive test. [2.40 (100 – 30)/100 = 1.68]. A dipstick method for diagnosis of malaria, which is highly sensitive and specific and is easily interpreted, is available at a cost of about US$1. If mefloquine is needed for treatment, it would be worthwhile using this test for diagnosis as long as the proportion of true cases remained below 58%. Similarly, in situations where artemisinin (Ct = US$1.50) is used for treatment, use of the dipstick test

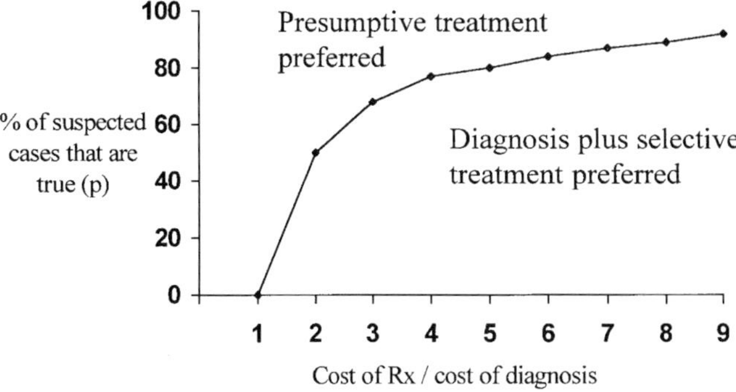

Figure 14.2 The relationship between costs of treatment in relation to the cost of diagnosis and the percentage of suspected cases that are true positives. Source: Phillips and Phillips-Howard, 1996

would be appropriate provided that the proportion of true cases was less than 33% (Phillips and Phillips-Howard, 1996). This relationship is illustrated in Figure 14.2.

A similar approach can be used in the case of tuberculosis. Assuming that treatment costs the health services US\$100, and that 50% of suspects have true TB, then the formula given above suggests that it would be reasonable to pay up to 100 × (100 − 50)/100 = US\$50 per diagnostic test. If only 20% of patients have TB but would none the less be put on TB treatment, detection cost could rise to US\$80 and still make economic sense. These figures do not take account of the public health impact of further transmission from cases who have presented for diagnosis but who have not been detected by microscopy.

Treatment

When a disease is highly prevalent a number of possible treatment strategies can be considered. The unlikely trio of schistosomiasis, onchocerciasis and STDs share the common property that variations on three possible treatment strategies—mass treatment versus screening and treatment versus treatment of individual cases—have all been tried. In the late 1980s, Prescott (1987) modelled four treatment strategies for schistosomiasis. These included two strategies without screening—mass population treatment and selected mass treatment (selection on the basis of age)—and two strategies with screening—screening and treatment of the entire population, and screening and treatment of a high-risk group, again selected on the basis of age. He found, not surprisingly, that the cost *per capita* rose as the fraction of the cases cured increased (Figure 14.3).

According to this model, the maximum expenditure of US\$1.70 yields a cure rate of about 72% of cases. If only US\$1 per person is available, the proportion of

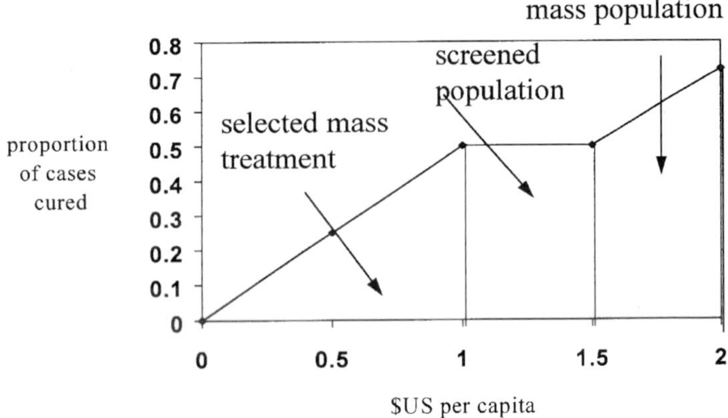

Figure 14.3 Costs *per capita* of various approaches to the treatment of tuberculosis. Source: Prescott, 1987

cases cured can attain about 50%. Interest in mass treatment of STDs has been fuelled by the HIV epidemic and more recently by the finding from the Mwanza Intervention study that syndromic treatment of STDs can lower HIV incidence by as much as 42% in a particular population. Since the majority of STDs are asymptomatic, this opens the question of what could be achieved in terms of slowing HIV transmission if *asymptomatic* cases could be treated effectively. This is being investigated in Rakai district of Uganda. It will be very interesting to compare the costs per HIV infection prevented of the Mwanza study, which used syndromic treatment of clinical cases, the Rakai mass treatment study, and of a third trial which is being carried out in neighbouring Masaka district of south-western Uganda, which involves the addition of health education and information, education and communication (IEC) to syndromic treatment of STDs.

Another issue of major concern is that of resistance to cheap first-line drugs. When is it appropriate to use a more effective but more expensive drug? Phillips and Phillips-Howard (1996), drawing on the example of antimalarials, have provided guidance on this issue also. The formula they propose is $Cf(F1 - F2) > Ct2 - Ct1$ where $Cf =$ the cost of failure, $F1$ and $F2$ are the failure rates of drugs 1 and 2, and $Ct1$ and $Ct2$ are the costs of treatment with drugs 1 and 2 respectively. Consideration of the implications of increasing resistance to the antimalarial drug sulphadoxine/pyrimethamine provides an example of this approach. Consider the situation in which the failure rate with sulfadoxine/pyrimethamine ($Ct1 =$ US$0.20) has reached 20%, and in which each failure gives rise to a cost of US$10 in lost wages, revisits and additional treatments, increased risk of death, disability, anaemia, etc. The alternative drug available is mefloquine at a cost of US$2.40, but with a high success rate of 97%. In this case it would not be worth shifting to the new drug since $Cf\,(F1 - F2)$ [$10 \times 17/100 = 1.70$] is less than

$Ct2 - Ct1$ (US\$2.20). When the percentage of failures with sulfadoxine/pyrimethamine rises to 25%, or the cost of mefloquine falls to US\$1.90, a change would make sense. This analysis is highly dependent on the 'cost of failure'; establishing this figure is difficult to do with precision. This type of calculation could be used in decisions about other drug combinations for TB, STDs and other infectious disease.

WHO now advocates strongly the DOTS (directly observed therapy short course) strategy for the treatment of tuberculosis. While in principle this strategy has much to recommend it, two aspects are of concern. First, it places an increased financial and economic burden not only on the health services, but also on patients in terms of time lost, travel costs, inconvenience and stigma. The DOTS strategy can be quite humiliating for a patient. In my view, the problems of this strategy have not been assessed objectively or acknowledged, and the economic work which has been commissioned to support it was geared to demonstrate the advantages and to minimise the problems of this approach to treatment. The second area of concern about DOTS is that it assumes implicitly that the patient is always responsible for failure to comply. In my experience, it is often the health services and not the patient that are non-compliant because drugs are not available. Perhaps DOTS will help in establishing a contract between the health services and the patients which makes it quite obvious when it is the health services, and not the patients, who are to blame for treatment failures.

Asking the right questions—the big picture

So far this paper has concentrated on decisions that need to be made at each step in the management of an infection, but a broader view is needed. It is possible to become lost in the details of the tradeoff between a 75% effective drug and a 99% effective drug when this may not be the main issue. Applying the Piot model to STDs gives a startling picture (Figure 14.4).

Data show that only about 7% of women who have a laboratory-confirmed STD receive appropriate care. Thus improvements in the process of treatment—even to the level of 100% efficacy—will have little effect on overall morbidity from STDs. Where should the economic emphasis be placed? How much would it cost to improve treatment-seeking behaviour, for example, to raise the fraction who seek care from a paltry 11%, and how much additional treatment cost would result? What should be done about the large fraction of asymptomatic infections? It is easy to worry about the fine-tuning of programmes and to lose sight of the main issue.

Finally, a few words about BSE. What would it have been worth spending early in the epidemic to try to detect BSE in the cattle? Expenditure on the epidemic so far has reached an estimated £1.5–2 bn—and if cases of nvCJD continue to occur there is no way of telling how high this might rise. Only a small fraction of this expenditure has gone on research.

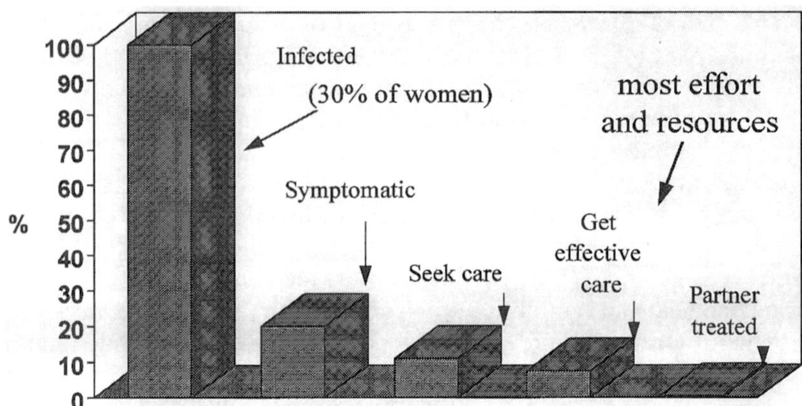

Figure 14.4 The pattern of STDs in Rakai District, Uganda. (Data from L. Paxton, Rakai Project, Uganda, 1997, personal communication)

About 9.5% of the UK herd of 10 million cattle have been infected with BSE, and 166 000 cases have been declared. If a way had been found to detect BSE, so allowing infected cattle to be removed from the herd thus preventing the possible transmission of BSE to humans, and assuming that two-thirds of the losses to the beef industry could have been averted, then the Phillips and Phillips-Howard's formula indicates that it would have been worth paying up to £120 per head to detect BSE in live cattle.

A major policy issue facing disease control is how crucial issues can be brought to the attention of those in a position to take appropriate steps, *early enough* in the epidemic for it to be useful. I suggest that economics, allied with public health epidemiology, has much to contribute to this effort.

References

Brinkmann U, Brinkmann A. Malaria and health in Africa: the present situation and epidemiological trends. *Tropical Medicine and Parasitology*, 1991; **42**: 204–213

Foster SD, Godfrey-Faussett P, Porter J. Modelling the economic benefits of tuberculosis preventive therapy for people with HIV: the example of Zambia. *AIDS*, 1997; **11**: 919–925

Najera JA, Liese BH, Hammer J. Malaria: new patterns and perspectives. Washington, DC: World Bank Technical Paper no 183, 1992

Needham D, Godfrey-Faussett P, Foster SD. Barriers to tuberculosis control in urban Zambia: the economic impact and burden on patients prior to diagnosis. Submitted for publication

Phillips M, Phillips-Howard P. Economic implications of resistance to antimalarial drugs. *Pharmacoeconomics*, 1996; **10**: 225–238

Prescott NM. The economics of schistosomiasis chemotherapy. *Parasitology Today*, 1987; **3**: 21–24

Saunderson PR. An economic evaluation of alternative programme designs for tuberculosis control in rural Uganda. *Social Science and Medicine*, 1995; **40**: 1203–1212

World Bank. *World Development Report*, 1993: *Investing in Health.* Washington, DC: Oxford University Press, 1993

15
The public health response to emerging infectious diseases: are current approaches adequate?

Ruth L. Berkelman

National Center for Infectious Diseases, Centers for Disease Control and Prevention, and Rollins School of Public Health, Emory University, Atlanta, USA

The emergence of AIDS towards the end of the 20th century came as an unexpected blow to medicine, public health and society (Figure 15.1). Facing up to the fact that the world was being confronted by a new and fatal infectious disease that was not only intensifying but also spreading globally was difficult and almost incomprehensible to many. Joshua Lederberg noted perceptively that a striking novelty of the late 20th century was the expectation in the developed countries of the world of near-perfect protection from contagious disease (Lederberg, 1992). Lewis Thomas stated that 'modern medicine has left on the public mind the conviction that we know almost everything about everything' (Thomas, 1992). It took almost a decade from the first recognition of AIDS for many public health professionals to put this disease into the overall context of emergence of infectious diseases.

Increased life expectancy in the late 19th and early 20th century can be attributed largely to improved sanitation, better nutrition, and less crowded living quarters—a higher standard of living combined with public health measures. The development of vaccines and antibiotics has also been tremendously useful. Yet, even today, there is still much to be learnt about infectious disease and a tremendous need for public health to remain vigorous.

New and Resurgent Infections: Prediction, Detection and Management of Tomorrow's Epidemics.
Edited by B. Greenwood and K. De Cock. Published 1998 John Wiley & Sons Ltd.

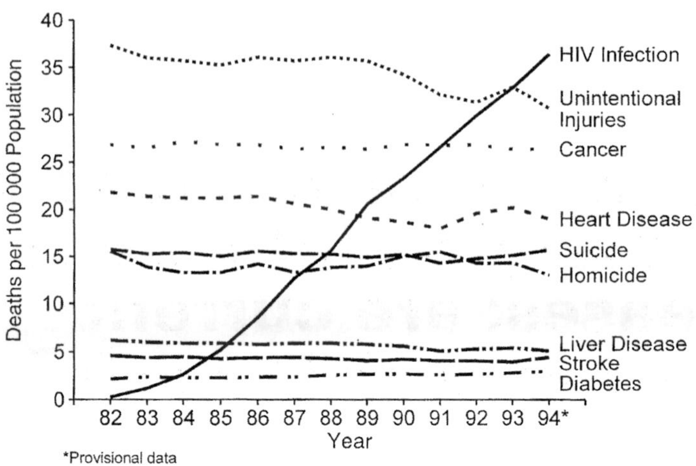

Figure 15.1 Death rates from leading causes of death in persons aged 25 to 44 years, USA, 1982–1994. Source: National Vital Statistics

Emerging infections: background

In the autumn of 1992, *Microbial Threats to Health: Emerging Infections* was published for the US Institute of Medicine (IOM) (Lederberg *et al*, 1992). The report stated that the USA and other parts of the world were vulnerable to both new and old microbial threats, and that much of this vulnerability was unnecessary. The report's recommendations did not attempt to address factors important to the emergence of infectious diseases such as population control, major societal changes (e.g. use of child care facilities, frequency of air travel), global climate change and land-use patterns. Instead, the recommendations focused on the critical need to strengthen the public health infrastructure to be better prepared to meet the challenges ahead. The report aimed many of its recommendations at the Centers for Disease Control and Prevention (CDC), and CDC began to draft a response within a month of publication of the IOM report.

At the same time as the IOM report was released, an article entitled 'Crisis in the hot zone' was published in *The New Yorker* (Preston, 1992). This article detailed the horror of Ebola haemorrhagic fever and then described the importation of Ebola virus into the USA via non-human primates. Soon afterwards, three major outbreaks occurred in the USA in quick succession: more than 50 children were hospitalized with acute renal failure after eating hamburger contaminated with *Escherichia coli* 0157:*H7*; 400 000 persons became ill with cryptosporidiosis in Milwaukee, Wisconsin after drinking contaminated municipal water; and more than 40 deaths were recorded among previously healthy young adults following infection with a newly recognized hantavirus harboured in deer mice (Berkelman, 1994). Each outbreak resulted in headlines in the national media, and media attention four years after release of the IOM report remains high and has become worldwide. Each real or perceived threat has generated an opportunity for scientists to explain to the public the problem and the proposed solution. Both media coverage and the publication of non-fiction books on the subject of emerging infections have generated immense public support for public health protection in the area of infectious diseases in the USA.

Addressing emerging infectious diseases: surveillance

CDC's plan *Addressing Emerging Infectious Diseases: A Prevention Strategy for the United States* was published in April 1994 after extensive internal and external review (CDC, 1994). Congressional appropriations to implement the CDC plan have increased each year since 1994 and total US$44.1 million for the fiscal year 1997. (Full implementation of the plan has been estimated to cost US$125 million annually.) Implementation of both the domestic and international components of the plan is well under way. Three major efforts have begun to improve surveillance and response domestically in the USA: strengthening state health department efforts in surveillance and response, developing sentinel physician networks, and initiating population-based programmes to address emerging infections (Berkelman *et al*, 1996).

First, federal resources have been devoted to strengthening the general system of disease detection and response activities, including laboratory investigation. The USA has relied for many decades on a system of disease notification. States determine which diseases must be reported by physicians and laboratories and together decide which diseases will be reported voluntarily by all states to the federal government each week. There are approximately 40 nationally notifiable diseases and, in the past few years, several have been added to the lists: *E. coli* 0157:*H*7, cryptosporidiosis, hantavirus pulmonary syndrome, invasive group A streptococcal infections, and invasive infections caused by drug-resistant *Streptococcus pneumoniae* (CDC, 1996a; 1997a). Depending on the disease, some states require that laboratory isolates be sent to the state laboratory; further analyses of isolates (e.g. *Salmonella* and *Neisseria meningitidis*) are often conducted in local or state public health laboratories.

In some states, additional personnel are being hired to strengthen the state's capacity to work closely with the medical community and to respond to reports of disease. Some resources are being used to initiate electronic reporting from commercial laboratories. Additionally, the new resources are strengthening the public health laboratory and, in some states, are allowing new molecular techniques to be used for epidemiological purposes. For example, use of pulsed-field gel electrophoresis to study *E. coli* 0157:*H*7 isolates helps to determine whether reported cases are the result of exposure to a common source, or whether they are sporadic.

In addition to strengthening surveillance and response capacity in state and

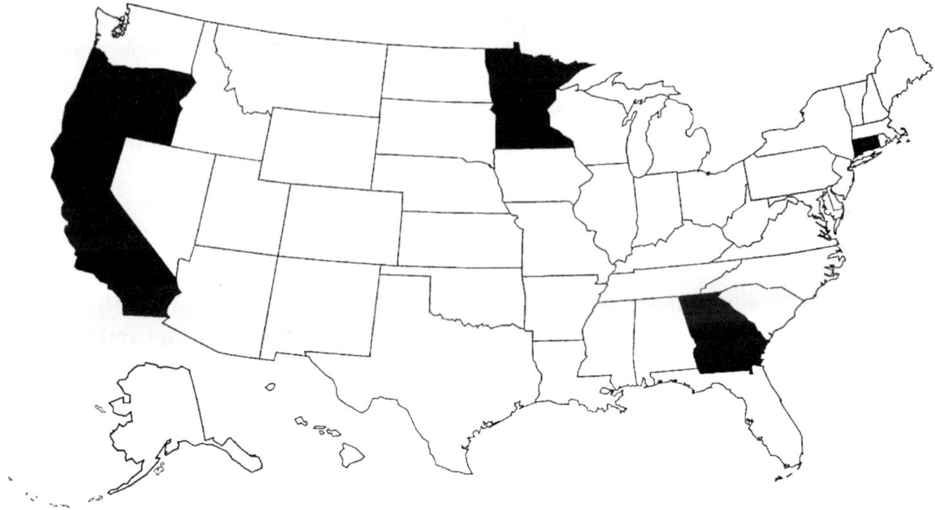

Figure 15.2 Emerging Infections Programmes, USA, 1996

local health departments, a second way in which CDC is strengthening surveillance is by improving current sentinel surveillance networks and initiating a few new ones. The new ones include a group of travel medicine clinics, a group of academically affiliated emergency departments, and a network of several hundred physicians who are members of the Infectious Diseases Society of America. For example, in emergency clinics, patients presenting with their first seizure are being tested for neurocysticercosis. As a result of travel to Central and South America, where cysticercosis is endemic, and of immigration from those areas, neurocysticercosis appears to be increasing in the USA (White, 1997). Europe has relied on reporting by networks of sentinel physicians for many years, and their usefulness has been documented in many settings (Stroobant *et al*, 1988).

Third, population-based emerging infections programmes (EIPs) have been developed in five states (California, Connecticut, Georgia, Minnesota, Oregon), covering together a total population of 16.9 million (Figure 15.2). These programmes are conducting intensive surveillance for, and research on, a number of diseases for which national data are limited. Additional programmes are being initiated in Maryland and New York. EIPs are based in state departments of public health and are led by epidemiologists; all are involved with partnerships in the community. In some settings, schools of medicine and/or schools of public health are involved; in other programmes, the primary partners are practitioners of infection control. The programmes are resource-intensive, but they have already proved to be quite useful at both local and national levels.

All five EIPs are determining the incidence of invasive infections caused by group A *Streptococcus*, group B *Streptococcus*, *Haemophilus influenzae* type *b*, drug-resistant *S. pneumoniae*, and *N. meningitidis* (Berkelman *et al*, 1996). Isolates are obtained to determine their resistance patterns, and molecular epidemiological tools are applied when appropriate. The US Department of Agriculture (USDA) and the Food and Drug Administration (FDA) are also collaborating with CDC and the EIPs to establish surveillance for food-borne diseases at these five sites (CDC, 1997b; Stephenson, 1997).

The EIPs have demonstrated flexibility in responding to new issues. When the UK reported 10 cases of variant Creutzfeldt–Jakob disease (CJD), potentially associated with the epidemic in cattle of bovine spongiform encephalopathy, the assistance of the EIPs was sought. Active surveillance in these sites for CJD, together with neuropathological examination, did not reveal any cases of the variant CJD, nor an unusual number of cases of CJD in young adults (CDC, 1996b).

Many epidemiologists are interested in devising a system for detection of an emerging pathogen, such as human immunodeficiency virus, *Legionella* or hepatitis C, in the absence of a tight clustering of cases in time and space. For example, thousands of deaths may have occurred in the USA from *Legionella* before the pathogen was recognised; earlier identification of the pathogen would have helped patient care. In response to this need for earlier alerts to the emergence of a virulent pathogen, four EIP sites are conducting surveillance for unexplained deaths and serious illnesses, possibly due to infectious causes (Perkins *et al*, 1996). Persons aged 1 to 49 years are eligible for investigation in three sites; in Oregon, the study is restricted to persons aged 1 to 39 years. Cases are reported by physicians, medical examiners, infection control practitioners and others. Surveillance personnel retrieve limited epidemiological and clinical data and store available clinical specimens. A copy of the medical record is also archived. After decisions are made regarding a ‘first round’ of laboratory testing, consideration is given to a ‘second round’ using research-level techniques such as universal nucleic acid primers.

As of March 1997, the illnesses of 76 individuals, including 25 who have died, are being investigated at these four sites. Preliminary data indicate that the most common primary syndromes were respiratory (31), neurological (13), cardiac (13), and multisystem organ failure (10) (Bradley Perkins, CDC, unpublished data). In many cases, specimens are unavailable. Limited laboratory testing at CDC has revealed a probable or definite diagnosis in a handful of cases: meningococcal disease, chlamydia, mycoplasma, and toxic shock syndrome are likely in at least one case. Although the project is complex and has not yet resulted in the identification of new infectious diseases, it has been useful in assessing the epidemiology of unexplained deaths and in identifying known infectious diseases for which the diagnosis is difficult or infrequently considered. Initiation of this project has resulted in a greater preparedness to address future outbreaks of severe or fatal illness of unknown aetiology.

Research

Both research and control efforts are also under way in these EIPs. For example, in Oregon, the incidence of meningococcal disease has increased steeply in recent years, with rates five-fold higher than in the rest of the USA (CDC, 1995). This increase has been largely the result of the appearance of serogroup B meningococcal strains belonging to the ET-5 complex. These ET-5 complex strains have been responsible for major epidemics in Norway, Iceland, Cuba and South America over the past 20 years. Research associated with Oregon's EIP has demonstrated that capsular switching may occur between virulent clones of meningococci, resulting in the escape of vaccine-induced or natural protective immunity. In the Oregon case, capsular switching from serogroup B to serogroup C occurred, a finding which may have important implications for vaccination against the disease (Swartley *et al*, 1997). An additional finding by the Oregon EIP that passive smoking is associated with an increased risk of meningococcal disease is being used to support efforts to prevent smoking (Fischer *et al*, 1997).

The development of diagnostic tests that are accurate and practical for field use was also targeted in the CDC plan. Research on diagnostic tests for tuberculosis, plague and sexually transmitted diseases is receiving renewed attention, with application of the molecular technology gains of the past decade being considered. One outstanding example of a diagnostic improvement is the use of immunohistochemical tests on skin biopsy specimens for the diagnosis of Ebola haemorrhagic fever (Zaki and Kilmarx, 1997). Skin biopsies can be performed easily in the most basic field conditions, and the formalin-fixed biopsy specimens are not infectious and can be transported without special precautions or refrigeration. This approach has advantages over viral cultures and fluorescent antibody tests which are commonly used for surveillance purposes, for samples used in these tests require special handling and a cold chain. The immunohistochemical findings have also provided new insights into the potential for transmission by contact.

In 1995, CDC reinstated an extramural research programme, which had ceased in 1973. Antibiotic resistance (e.g. determining methods to reduce inappropriate use of antibiotics) and tick-borne diseases (e.g. defining the ecology of ehrlichiosis) are areas of research that have been targeted for inclusion in the initial implementation of this programme.

International collaboration

CDC contributes to the efforts which are under way internationally to address the problem of emerging infectious diseases. CDC has strengthened the approximately 25 WHO collaborating centres based at CDC (WHO maintains approximately 1200 collaborating centres worldwide). One impetus for reviewing these centres was the recognition, following the outbreak of plague in India, that CDC's plague activities needed strengthening, and that other collaborating centres might also need improvements. Therefore, CDC evaluated each of its collaborating centres to determine whether the terms of reference were being met fully and whether their capabilities should be strengthened. As a result, CDC is in a far better position to support the WHO and others requiring assistance from the USA in a number of disease areas such as cholera, plague, malaria, and rickettsial diseases. In addition, a collaborating centre for food-borne diseases has recently been initiated.

CDC has also assisted WHO with strengthening specific networks such as the one for arboviruses and viral haemorrhagic fevers. Arbovirus outbreaks are common, their biology is complex, and their diagnosis is difficult, with over 500 arboviruses registered worldwide. Networks for such diseases demand continuing attention. Many of the laboratories in the network had originally been supported by the Rockefeller Foundation, including those in Brazil, Nigeria, southern Africa, India and the USA, but outside support to these laboratories ceased more than a decade ago (James LeDuc, personal communication). The laboratories have had to function with whatever resources were available in their countries (James LeDuc, personal communication). In 1993, WHO surveyed 34 virology laboratories that are used as reference centres (LeDuc, 1996). The survey determined that approximately half of these laboratories lacked the ability to diagnose diseases such as yellow fever, hantavirus pulmonary syndrome and Rift Valley fever, often because they lacked diagnostic reagents. With a relatively small infusion of resources, diagnostic reagents for yellow fever, hantavirus and dengue have been distributed to some of these laboratories. Opening channels of communication has also helped to revitalise this network. CDC co-sponsored a meeting with WHO of the directors of the collaborating centres; it was their first meeting together in over a decade.

CDC is also working with WHO in individual countries. In 1992, Kenya experienced its first outbreak of yellow fever in decades; in 1994, two technologists from the Kenya Medical Research Institute (KEMRI) received extensive training at CDC's laboratories as part of KEMRI's efforts to develop a regional reference centre for yellow fever and to build on its sentinel surveillance system for yellow fever in Kenya (Sanders *et al*, 1996). In 1995, CDC worked with WHO to support a workshop in yellow fever diagnosis held at KEMRI, a meeting which two individuals from each of several neighbouring East African countries attended. Although relatively small in scope and requiring limited resources, such steps are useful as building blocks in ensuring that the necessary infrastructure for surveillance exists regionally.

In the USA, other agencies have also been tackling the issue of emerging infections. The National Institute of Allergy and Infectious Diseases has developed a research agenda for emerging infectious diseases (US National Institutes of Health, 1996) and the Fogarty International Center of the National Institutes of Health (NIH) has developed a training programme in emerging infections for scientists from developing countries. In addition, a working group

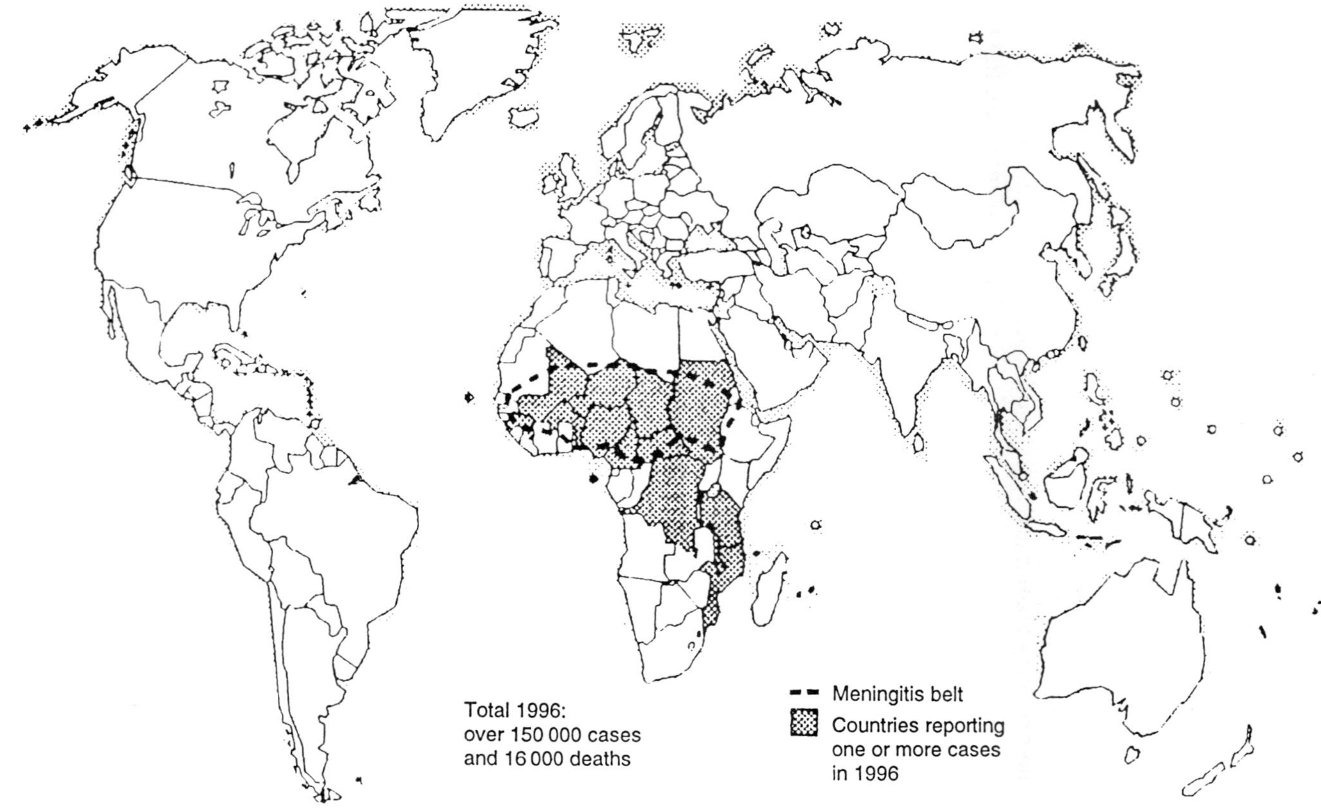

Figure 15.3 Epidemic meningitis in Africa, 1996 and 'meningitis belt'

and task force on emerging infections has been organised with representatives from 17 federal agencies, including CDC, the Department of Defense, FDA, NIH, and USDA (US National Science and Technology Council, 1995). An effort to address international threats more comprehensively at the federal level was initiated by the Committee on International Science, Engineering and Technology (CISET).

Under the auspices of the task force, CDC has been working closely with WHO and its regional offices and other partners to build up a capacity to control meningitis outbreaks within 17 African countries (Figure 15.3). WHO's plan of action includes improving surveillance in these countries; three collaborating centres for reference and research on meningococci (France, Norway and US) are active partners in strengthening laboratory capability in these countries, including training, provision of reference services, diagnostic reagents and reference strains (WHO, 1997). Partners in this field include Medecins Sans Frontières, the International Federation of the Red Cross, UNICEF, and others. These partnerships are new, and some are unprecedented. The impression of scientists in the field is that communications are far better in many of these countries than in years past, that surveillance is working, that laboratories are available to confirm the disease, and that countries are more ready for public health action than they were during the 1996 epidemic of meningitis (Bradley Perkins, personal observation). In addition, the open communication facilitated by WHO may have prevented unnecessary stockpiling of vaccine by individual countries that may have led to depletion of reserves. These successes need to be documented, and weak links in the surveillance and response arms need to be strengthened.

The USA is also working on a US–European agenda, with a preliminary aim of co-operating to improve laboratories in Africa. A US–Japan agenda and a bilateral agreement with South Africa on emerging infectious diseases are currently being negotiated as well.

There is national and global interest in developing regional hubs of excellence in diagnosis and investigation of new and resurgent microbial threats. The South African Institute of Virology, the US Naval Medical Research Unit in Egypt, and KEMRI are examples of laboratories that have been proposed as potential regional resources for Africa.

Plans for emerging infectious diseases

Since 1992, many plans to address the problem of emerging infections have been developed by various governments and organisations. Canada (Canadian Expert Working Group on Emerging Infectious Disease Issues, 1994), WHO (1997) and several of WHO's regional offices have developed such plans. A European programme in epidemiology and response to emerging infections was initiated in 1995 (Giesecke, 1995). The European Union is sponsoring a two-year training programme, a programme which emphasizes the irrelevance of national boundaries in disease control efforts. SALM-Net and the surveillance network for Legionnaires' disease are excellent examples of European co-operation between countries, resulting in improved control of salmonellosis and Legionnaires' disease within the European Union, with benefits to other countries as well (Hutchinson *et al*, 1996; Joseph *et al*, 1996; Killalea *et al*, 1996). SALM-Net is currently being enhanced to include surveillance for *E. coli* O157:H7 and drug-resistant *Salmonella* isolates (Christopher Bartlett, personal communication).

Almost all plans to address emerging infections include three major elements: early detection and response, research, and implementation of measures of prevention. Critical to each of these elements is the necessary infrastructure, including the laboratory facilities, equipment, and trained personnel. Development plans also emphasize the critical role of partnerships, both with other countries and with non-governmental organizations. Finally, these plans recognize that even the soundest strategy cannot guarantee success, but all share the conviction that being prepared is the best means of protection.

Efforts at prevention are clearly in progress at all levels, covering an enormous number of opportunities. In the USA, educational activities aimed at the public have been initiated to promote appropriate antibiotic use, hand washing (Operation Clean Hands), and safe handling of fresh fruit and produce. Professional education has also been heightened, with efforts such as the initiation of the journal *Emerging Infectious Diseases*. Globally, the number of prevention activities, such as increasing vaccine use, ensuring safety of food and water supplies, and controlling disease vectors, is also growing, but these clearly require further investment. The steps taken to date are small ones in a lengthy journey.

Constraints

What are the threats to these expanding efforts to tackle emerging infectious diseases? Renewed efforts to address infectious diseases must be nurtured and valued by policy-makers, and protecting the population from large-scale infections must be recognized by all as an integral part of public health. Resources will be needed to make these efforts thrive and to cultivate the other activities that are needed.

Sometimes, unpopular decisions must be made to address microbial threats. For example, assuring rational use of antibiotics may require more than education. The growing problem of antimicrobial resistance for so many conditions may require consideration of measures that many would describe as draconian (e.g. restriction of the use of vancomycin, changes in the use of antimicrobial agents for veterinary use, and a decrease in the over-the-counter drug availability for human use).

Another contentious issue relates to a country's willingness to share information on its health problems with other countries (often referred to as 'transparency').

Economic risk is frequently cited as the reason a country may not report cases of a disease to WHO. At times, an economic risk exists, but this risk may be overestimated, and the potential economic gains that may accompany international assistance and greater accuracy in media reporting may be underestimated. As an example, India suffered an estimated two billion dollar economic loss in the wake of the plague epidemic in Surat following widespread hysteria out of proportion to the size of the outbreak (US National Science and Technology Council, 1995). Indeed, no cases were confirmed in any major city outside Surat, and dissemination of information based on accurate surveillance and diagnosis might have averted some of these losses.

A rumour of an outbreak may cause as much economic havoc as a true outbreak. It is reported that tourism at seaside resorts in Kenya fell off tremendously in June 1995 when a rumour of haemorrhagic fever in these areas reached the Italian press, even though no cases of haemorrhagic fever were confirmed (*Daily Nation*, 1995).

A country's ability to gain international assistance for a true outbreak or to obtain confirmation from an external organization of the absence of disease should be a tremendous asset. Circumstances in which reporting has helped a country either to confirm the absence of disease or to control the outbreak and address problems rapidly and effectively should be documented. A country will be most open if effective assistance can be guaranteed.

Complacency or neglect, civil strife and war all threaten and will continue to threaten the public health infrastructure. For many policymakers, control is dull and often requires a repetitive activity, such as vaccination of children. If a disease is seen rarely, surveillance systems may be allowed to erode. When a measles outbreak occurred in the USA in 1989–91, a tremendous effort was put into assuring appropriate vaccination of young children, and in 1993 a headline read '3 Years after an Epidemic, Measles is Called Defeated' (*New York Times*, 1993). Yet measles was not defeated; it was controlled, and, in the absence of eradication, measles will continue to be controlled in the USA and elsewhere only with continuing aggressive efforts to vaccinate children.

The failure to eradicate a disease that has been targeted for eradication may result in a greater degree of complacency towards control of that disease than was present before the eradication campaign started. Once a decision is made to eradicate a disease, such as the current programme to eradicate polio, full support is needed to ensure as great an opportunity for success as possible. When the malaria eradication campaign began to fail, an acceptable strategy for malaria control to replace efforts at eradication was difficult to define and to implement; in addition, the recognition that global malaria eradication may not be attainable led to withdrawal of financial support by many institutions (Najera, 1989). Malaria has subsequently re-emerged in many countries, with an added burden of increasing drug resistance.

Preparedness for the future

Recently there has been a major focus on the global burden of disease, and significant advances have been made in this arena, particularly the development of the concept of disability-adjusted life years (Murray, 1996). Knowledge of the current burden of morbidity and mortality may be extremely helpful in directing resources for implementation of major programmes of prevention. However, for infectious diseases, the potential burden of a disease may be as, or more, important than the current burden when needs for technical expertise (e.g. plague) and for surveillance and response capacity are assessed. In addition, issues like biological terrorism, xenotransplantation, or vancomycin-resistant *Staphylococcus aureus* may have caused little or no morbidity or mortality but still demand public health consideration.

Epidemiological and demographic transition theses have become important to public health policy-making in the past two decades (World Bank, 1993). The theses have been developed and tested primarily in the developed world; how well they will operate in parts of Africa, Indonesia, and other parts of the developing world is less well understood. For example, urbanization in the developed world has meant better sanitation and other amenities which favour a decline in infectious diseases; yet many of the megacities forecast to emerge in the next few decades will be in the developing world (Rousch, 1994) and are likely to include sprawling slums with high human density and poor housing and sanitation. The global burden of infectious diseases is projected to decline in the coming decades, but vigilance is warranted (Murray, 1996).

Finally, the ceaseless adaptation of microbes to their environment will continue to deal humanity its surprises, as in 1918–19, when pandemic influenza swept around the world causing an estimated 20 million deaths. Whether the appearance of a new pandemic strain of influenza, the emergence of *Vibrio cholerae* 0139, or the development of antimalarial drug resistance, each emerging or newly recognized disease should be investigated and a measured and rational response initiated.

An example of such disease emergence that requires investigation is the paramyxovirus recently recognized in Australia (Selvey *et al*, 1995). In 1994, in Brisbane, 21 horses were infected, of which 14 died or were euthanised after severe signs of an acute respiratory disease had developed; two persons were infected and one died. A smaller outbreak among horses with one human death occurred 1000 km from Brisbane a month later. The name 'equine morbillivirus' has been proposed for the paramyxovirus isolated from a human and four of the horses. Current evidence suggests that the reservoirs of the virus are fruit bats or flying foxes (Young *et al*, 1996). There has been no further occurrence of the disease, and the events may be considered a failed adaptation of the virus to the human species. The current efforts, including establishing surveillance for this disease, isolating the aetiological agent and determining the mode of transmission and the reservoirs of infection, are each important steps in preparing public health professionals to address future occurrences in human populations.

In a hypothetical scenario related to the year 2012, the virologist C. J. Peters contemplates the potential for this recently recognized paramyxovirus to emerge in the densely populated city of Bangkok (Peters and Olshaker, 1997). The city is described in conditions similar to those that prevail today in many large cities, with overcrowded, understaffed, and undersupplied clinics responsible for the problems of the poor. In such circumstances, cases of severe and frequently fatal respiratory illnesses may go undiagnosed for a lengthy period. Even when the Ministry of Health is alerted, lack of resources may slow its response. Investigation eventually demonstrates a 50% mortality rate and identifies the aetiology to be similar to the paramyxovirus seen in 1994. Three months after the doctor saw the first sick child, the disease has spread throughout the poorer sections of Bangkok, with pockets of infection exploding, particularly in massage parlours. These are spots frequently visited by tourists, and soon infected businessmen bring the disease home with them. When the epidemic grows so large that the news media pick it up, cases are linked worldwide.

The underlying issue in this scenario is not whether this particular virus will adapt to the human population and a worldwide outbreak occur, but rather that conditions exist to spawn such an outbreak and that there is a need to be prepared for such an event. Having recognized a highly fatal pathogen that may be transmitted through the respiratory route, public health professionals should consider what measures might be needed to control it, for example, development and dissemination of diagnostic tests, definition of the patterns of endemicity, and possible treatment options such as determining the efficacy of ribavirin in experimentally infected animals. If there were an outbreak in Bangkok, the scenarios that followed are likely to be quite different, depending on whether some minimum level of preparation had been accomplished.

Infectious diseases continue to demand enormous public health attention and will continue to do so in the future. The world is not in equilibrium, and we must be prepared for the inevitability of surprises. The human species will continue to be vulnerable to large-scale infections, and we must use our collective wits and resources to assure the best chances for a good outcome when these occur.

References

Berkelman RL. Emerging infectious diseases in the United States, 1993. *Journal of Infectious Diseases*, 1994; **170**: 272–277

Berkelman RL, Pinner RW, Hughes JM. Addressing emerging microbial threats in the United States. *Journal of the American Medical Association*, 1996; **275**: 315–317

Canadian Expert Working Group on Emerging Infectious Disease Issues. Proceedings and recommendations of the Expert Working Group on Emerging Infectious Disease Issues: Lac Tremblant declaration. *Canadian Communicable Disease Report*, 1994; **20** S2: 1–21

CDC. *Addressing Emerging Infectious Disease Threats: A Prevention Strategy for the United States*. Atlanta, GA: US Dept of Health and Human Services, Public Health Service, 1994

CDC. Serogroup B meningococcal disease—Oregon 1994. *Morbidity and Mortality Weekly Report*, 1995; **44**: 121–124

CDC. Surveillance for Creutzfeldt–Jacob disease—United States. *Morbidity and Mortality Weekly Report*, 1996a; **45**: 665–668

CDC. *MMWR Summary of Notifiable Disease, United States 1995*. Atlanta, GA: US Dept of Health and Human Services, Public Health Service, 1996b

CDC. Case definitions for infectious conditions under public health surveillance. *Morbidity and Mortality Weekly Report*, 1997a; **46**(RR-10): 1–56

CDC. Foodborne Diseases Active Surveillance Network, 1996. *Morbidity and Mortality Weekly Report*, 1997b; **46**: 258–261

Daily Nation. Hotel Bookings down by 40pc. 26 June 1995

Fischer M, Hedberg K, Cardosi P *et al.* Epidemic meningococcal disease and tobacco smoke: A risk factor study in the Pacific Northwest. *Paediatric Infectious Diseases*, 1997; **16**: 979–983

Giesecke J. Preparing Europe to deal with outbreaks. *Lancet*, 1995; **346**: 897

Hutchinson EJ, Joseph CA, Bartlett CLR on behalf of the Working Group for Legionella Infections. EWGLI: a European surveillance scheme for travel associated legionnaires' disease. *Eurosurveillance*, 1996; **1**: 37–39

Joseph C, Morgan D, Birtles R, Pelaz C *et al.* An international investigation of an outbreak of legionnaires' disease among UK and French tourists. *European Journal of Epidemiology*, 1996; **12**: 215–219

Killalea D, Ward LR, Roberts D *et al.* International epidemiological and microbiological study of outbreak of *Salmonella agona* infections from a ready to eat savoury snack. I. England and Wales and the United States. *British Medical Journal*, 1996; **313**: 1105–1107

Lederberg J. Pandemic as a natural evolutionary phenomenon. In: Mack A (ed), *In Time of Plague: The History and Consequences of Lethal Epidemic Disease*. New York: New York University Press, 1992, pp 21–38

Lederberg J, Shope RE, Oaks SC Jr (eds). *Emerging Infections: Microbial Threats to Health in the United States*. Washington, DC: National Academy Press, 1992

LeDuc JW. WHO program on emerging virus diseases. *Archives of Virology*, 1996; **11**(suppl): 13–20

Murray CJL, Lopez AD. *The Global Burden of Disease: A Comprehensive Assessment of Mortality and Disability from Diseases, Injuries and Risk Factors in 1990 and Projected to 2020*. Cambridge, MA: Harvard School of Public Health, 1996

Najera JA. Malaria and the work of WHO. *Bulletin of the World Health Organization*, 1989; **67**: 229–243

New York Times, 29 October 1993

Perkins BA, Flood JM, Danila R *et al.* Unexplained deaths due to possibly infectious causes in the United States: defining the problem and designing surveillance and laboratory approaches. The Unexplained Deaths Working Group. *Emerging Infectious Diseases*, 1996; **2**: 47–53

Peters CJ, Olshaker M. *Virus Hunter*. New York: Anchor Books, Doubleday, 1997

Preston R. Crisis in the hot zone. *The New Yorker*, 26 October 1992, pp 58–81

Roush W. Population: the view from Cairo. *Science*, 1994; **265**: 1164–1167

Sanders EJ, Borus P, Ademba G, Kuria G, Tukei PM, LeDuc JW. Sentinel surveillance for yellow fever in Kenya, 1993 to 1995. *Emerging Infectious Diseases*, 1996; **2**: 236–238

Selvey LA, Wells RM, McCormack JG *et al.* Infection of humans and horses by a newly described morbillivirus. *Medical Journal of Australia*, 1995; **162**: 642–645

Stephenson J. Public health experts take aim at a moving target: foodborne infections. *Journal of the American Medical Association*, 1997; **277**: 97–98

Stroobant A, Van Casteren V, Thiers G. Surveillance systems from primary-care data: surveillance through a network of sentinel general practitioners. In: Eylenbosch WJ, Noah ND (eds), *Surveillance in Health and Disease*. Oxford: Oxford University Press, 1988, pp 62–74

Swartley JS, Marfin AA, Edupuganti S *et al.* Capsule switching of *Neisseria meningitidis*. *Proceedings of the National Academy of Sciences of the USA*, 1997; **94**: 271–276

Thomas L. Science and health—possibilities, probabilities, and limitations. In: Mack A (ed), *In Time of Plague: The History and Social Consequences of Lethal Epidemic Disease*. New York: New York University Press, 1992, p 60

US National Institutes of Health. The NIAID research agenda for emerging infectious diseases. Bethesda, July 1996

US National Science and Technology Council. *Report of the Committee on International Science, Engineering and Technology Working Group on Emerging and Re-emerging Infectious Diseases: Infectious Disease—A Global Health Threat*, September 1995

White AC. Neurocysticercosis: a major cause of neurological disease worldwide. *Clinical Infectious Diseases*, 1997; **24**: 101–115

World Bank. *World Development Report* 1993: *Investing in Health*. Washington, DC: Oxford University Press, 1993

World Health Organization. *EMC Annual Report 1996*. Geneva: World Health Organization, 1997

Young PL, Halpin K, Selleck PW *et al.* Serologic evidence for the presence in Pteropus bats of a paramyxovirus related to equine morbillivirus. *Emerging Infectious Diseases*, 1996; **2**: 239–240

Zaki SR, Kilmarx P. Ebola virus hemorrhagic fever. In: Horsburgh CR, Nelson AM (eds), *Pathology of Emerging Infections: A Clinical and Pathological Update*. Washington, DC: American Society for Microbiology Press, 1997

16
Emerging diseases: a global response to a global challenge

Lindsay J. Martinez and David L. Heymann

Division of Emerging and other Communicable Diseases Surveillance and Control, World Health Organization, Geneva, Switzerland

Although advances in public health and medicine, sanitation and pest control have led to the prevention and control of communicable diseases in some countries, such advances have had minimal impact in many others. Worldwide, gains have been undermined to various degrees by deteriorating public health infrastructures, under-resourced health care services, and the rise of new and multidrug-resistant organisms.

In the past decade, the world has had to cope with an impressive array of emergent or resurgent infectious diseases while continuing to battle against common and known diseases. Today the potential for localized diseases quickly to become global public health hazards is enhanced by the increasing volume of international travel and the worldwide expansion of trade. Demographic growth, migration and uncontrolled urbanization, poverty, changes in human behaviour, and changes in land use and environment all contribute to the remarkable persistence of many communicable diseases.

WHO's response

Recognising these recent developments, the Member States of WHO called upon the Organization to strengthen and coordinate global surveillance and control of communicable diseases in a resolution adopted in 1995. In response to this resolution, the Division of Emerging and other Communicable Diseases (EMC) was established in October 1995 to bring together WHO's existing surveillance activities, to promote the development of national and international infrastructure and resources to recognize, monitor and respond to communicable diseases and

New and Resurgent Infections: Prediction, Detection and Management of Tomorrow's Epidemics.
Edited by B. Greenwood and K. De Cock.

emerging health problems. Within this mandate, WHO seeks to facilitate and coordinate communicable disease surveillance and responses to outbreaks and epidemics.

WHO is reshaping and strengthening a global network for disease surveillance. This network will be the basis for rapid and effective mobilization of control measures. Its global scope is essential since communicable diseases do not respect national or regional boundaries; a disease outbreak may have its origin in a distant country, and even localized outbreaks can have major international and economic repercussions (e.g. plague in India in 1994, Ebola haemorrhagic fever in Zaire in 1995, new variant CJD in the UK in 1996). The role of WHO will be to provide this network with common terminology and common case definitions, thus facilitating international comparison of epidemiological data. At the same time, WHO is promoting prompt and transparent case reporting and transmission of epidemiological information. A common policy framework is provided through the International Health Regulations.

Building on success

Despite the heavy burden of communicable disease that persists today, notably in developing countries, there have been important successes in WHO's efforts to alleviate the problem. WHO has achieved the eradication of smallpox and has brought a number of other diseases (polio, dracunculiasis, leprosy, Chagas disease) to the point where eradication or elimination is now within sight, and great progress has been made in controlling others, such as measles and neonatal tetanus. A major achievement has been the elimination of onchocerciasis (river blindness) as a public health problem from 11 countries in West Africa. Influenza surveillance is a long-standing priority of WHO, involving a worldwide network of laboratories generating data that enable WHO to recommend each year the composition of the next season's influenza vaccine. No other organization has this experience and expertise in the international surveillance and control of communicable diseases.

Networking

WHO has long-standing experience in the promotion of international collaboration and research through its networks of Collaborating Centres. These Centres are selected on the basis of excellence in specialized areas and carry out specific activities on behalf of WHO. Activities include laboratory diagnosis, production and supply of diagnostic reagents, specialized training, technical advice and support to developing countries. To increase geographic representation, more centres are being established in developing countries, with an emphasis on training needs and laboratory support. An assessment of the existing Centres is under way, in order better to define their capabilities and needs.

The Collaborating Centres are involved in many active surveillance programmes, collecting information on diseases such as influenza, arbovirus diseases and haemorrhagic fevers, hepatitis, poliomyelitis, HIV/AIDS, tuberculosis, malaria, zoonoses and food-borne diseases. Surveillance of antimicrobial resistance is being strengthened with the development of a global network of laboratories providing quality-controlled data. Global surveillance of Creutzfeldt–Jakob disease is now being organized.

Global information systems utilize up-to-date communication technologies to ensure that information collected through global monitoring is rapidly and widely disseminated. EMC is now linking its Collaborating Centres and other institutions electronically to form a global information system for disease monitoring and control.

Sources of information available from EMC include:

- News on disease outbreaks and WHO interventions, updated as information becomes available, are posted on EMC's home page on the World Wide Web (WWW) and provided by electronic mail to the general public. A restricted system, available to Ministries of Health and Collaborating Centres, shares information on rumours of outbreaks and the WHO action being taken to investigate them.
- *The Weekly Epidemiological Record* (WER) reports on the diseases coming within the provisions of the International Health Regulations (i.e. plague, cholera and yellow fever) as well as providing information on outbreaks, progress in controlling diseases to be eradicated/eliminated (polio, leprosy, dracunculiasis) and other news of public health importance relating to communicable diseases. The WER is now available electronically.

Being better prepared

Preparedness for communicable disease prevention and control is a primary goal of EMC. Achieving this requires a substantial and long-term commitment of human and material resources to strengthen the infrastructure and processes for disease surveillance and control.

Surveillance is at the heart of national infectious disease control programmes. Relevant, accurate and timely information can avert a local or national outbreak and, at the same time, prevent a crisis at the international level. Strong surveillance and control systems help to identify areas of high risk for disease, guide immunization and prevention strategies, and detect and control the re-emergence of disease within a country. To strengthen the national and international infrastructure necessary to recognize, report and respond to communicable diseases, EMC provides technical guidance on international consensus policies on surveillance and control strategies, facilitates activities of governments and non-governmental organizations in the training of epidemiologists and public health specialists, and solicits government support for these efforts.

The many activities and linkages in this area illustrate the need for a strong, coordinated and engaged system at the international level, while national and regional systems improve their capacities. The prevention of communicable and zoonotic diseases, including those diseases with epidemic potential, requires long-term, multi-sectoral commitment to the creation and maintenance of an infrastructure to monitor and respond. To be sustainable, this must eventually be fully integrated with national health, sanitation and communications systems.

Responding to outbreaks

WHO now intervenes more directly than in the past in outbreaks and epidemics. At the request of the country concerned, a team will arrive on site within 24 hours to make an initial evaluation. This is possible because of WHO's use of *laissez-passer* and its access to accelerated visa and travel formalities. After this initial response, EMC arranges intervention as required from international partners, including personnel and supplies, operational support and resource mobilization. The full international team ensures a complete investigation of the epidemic, organizes and assists in implementing appropriate control measures, assesses needs for supplies and equipment, provides training to local personnel and educational information to the public and plans follow-up activities.

A common code of practice

The International Health Regulations (IHR) constitute a unique universal health convention, providing an internationally agreed code of practice for controlling the international spread of potentially dangerous infectious diseases. Under the present version of the IHR, measures apply specifically to plague, cholera and yellow fever, for which reporting is mandatory. However, countries often fear the stigma and economic consequences associated with these diseases, and are reluctant to report. The IHR are based on the principle of maximum security with minimum interference in traffic and trade, and stipulate the maximum permitted measures to be taken. Since the IHR were adopted in 1969, there have been major changes in disease epidemiology together with massive increases in international travel and trade. In a resolution adopted in 1995, the World Health Assembly called for revision of the IHR to make them more applicable to the control of communicable diseases in the 21st century. WHO is now organizing this revision. The objective is to devise IHR which will provide a valuable public health tool and assist through improved reporting in strengthening the global alert and response to outbreaks of diseases likely to trigger international action.

Looking ahead

WHO, through the activities of EMC, is strengthening international surveillance and reporting of communicable diseases. Networks of Collaborating Centres are being evaluated, extended and strengthened as necessary. A suite of accessible and affordable electronic communications will be exploited to increase and accelerate effective information exchange. The ability of countries to recognize and respond quickly to disease outbreaks will be enhanced, assisted as needed by WHO and its networks of Collaborating Centres, so that they are rapidly contained at the source of the infection. Updated IHR will provide a legal framework and common policy to assist public health officials in dealing with outbreaks and epidemics. EMC's vision for the 21st century is a world on the alert and able to contain communicable diseases through:

- strong national disease surveillance and control programmes;
- global networks of centres, organizations and individuals to monitor diseases;
- rapid information exchange through electronic links; and
- effective national and international preparedness, and rapid response to contain epidemics of international importance.

17
Emerging infectious diseases: setting the research and public health agenda

Brian Greenwood

Department of Infectious and Tropical Diseases, London School of Hygiene & Tropical Medicine, UK

During the past few years emerging and resurgent infections have received substantial attention in both the medical and the general press. Outbreaks of exotic and fatal diseases, such as Ebola virus infection and pneumonic plague, appeal to the public's interest in both medical matters and disasters in a way that has been exploited fully by the media. Research scientists have also been quick to exploit this reawakening of public concern with infectious diseases, persuading several of the major research donors to increase their support for research in the area of emerging infections. Has this been just self-serving or is the increased attention now been given to emerging and resurgent infections by the international health community fully justified? The papers presented during the course of the Forum strongly support the latter view.

Papers presented elsewhere in this volume (Epstein, chapter 3; Anthony J. McMichael, chapter 2) have reviewed ways in which some of the major changes in human society and behaviour that have taken place during the past ten thousand years, such as the establishment of settled agriculture, domestication of animals, urbanization and industrialization, have provided new opportunities for microbes that they have exploited fully; there is nothing new in the concept of emerging infections. However, it seems likely that this process has been accelerated by the major environmental and social changes that have taken place during the past two hundred years. A massive increase in population, increased opportunities for travel, accelerated urbanization with the establishment of megacities, pollution,

New and Resurgent Infections: Prediction, Detection and Management of Tomorrow's Epidemics.
Edited by B. Greenwood and K. De Cock.

exploitation of virgin lands, changes in agricultural practices, global warming and changes in sexual behaviour are some of the processes discussed during the Forum which have each contributed to the emergence of new infections or to the resurgence of old ones during the past few decades (Bradley, this volume, chapter 1; Gubler, this volume, chapter 9; Kestens and Vanham, this volume, chapter 6).

The development of effective vaccines against the common diseases of childhood, such as measles, and the discovery of antibiotics were major factors that led to the complacency about infectious diseases that was prevalent in the industrialized world 20 years ago. However, many pathogens of humans have a remarkable ability to respond to external stresses, through mutation or genetic recombination, and their potential to develop resistance to antibiotics and to vaccine-induced immune responses was underestimated seriously. The ability of the HIV virus to vary most of its genome every few days and the implications of this plasticity for vaccine development are discussed earlier in this volume (Andrew McMichael, chapter 4). Levin (this volume, chapter 5) pointed out how antibiotic-resistant bacteria may prevail even when not exposed to heavy drug pressure because of the occurrence of additional mutations. At present, several important human pathogens are developing drug resistance at a faster rate than the pharmaceutical industry can develop new drugs to which they are sensitive. The problem of resurgent, drug-resistant infections is a real one.

How should the public health community respond to this threat? In the short term, emphasis must be placed on surveillance and prompt responses to outbreaks. In the longer term, it may be possible to influence some of the processes that underlie the recent increase in emerging and re-emerging infections, but this will be difficult.

Surveillance

Surveillance is critical to the problem of new and resurgent infections but it is not easy to achieve. Effective surveillance requires collection of relevant and reliable field data, rapid transfer of these data to a central co-ordinating centre where they can be compiled, and correct interpretation of the collated results.

In most industrialized countries, reporting of serious infectious diseases is mandatory, allowing the rapid compilation of regional and national statistics and early detection of changes in the incidence of infections such as meningitis, even if some under-reporting occurs. Advances in computerization have facilitated the management of these large data sets. Unfortunately, the situation in many developing countries is very different. Although routine reporting of infectious diseases is often undertaken, the quality of the data collected is very variable. Clinical diagnoses are only rarely supported by microbiological diagnosis, systems for the transfer of data to a regional centre are lacking, compilation of data is frequently delayed and the motivation of staff is low because they rarely see any response to their reporting activities. Two ways of improving this situation are being followed—overall improvement of routine surveillance systems and the establishment of focal surveillance sites.

Developments in computerization, for example access to satellite transmission systems, provide one route for the improvement of general reporting schemes. Simple computerization of reports and electronic transfer of data provide both a means for the speedy transfer of routine statistics from the field to a regional centre and, equally importantly, a route for the rapid return of collated information to those working in the field together with suggestions as to how this information could be used. In areas with limited resources, microbiological diagnosis is likely to remain a problem, but at least data management can be improved relatively cheaply using modern methods of communication.

Identification of focal sites where high-quality data are collected routinely is an old idea which, in some circumstances, has proved to be very effective. Thus, the WHO-supported global influenza virus surveillance system has provided important guidelines to the manufacturers of influenza vaccines for many years. WHO is currently strengthening its network of surveillance laboratories in Africa and in other parts of the developing world (LeDuc, 1996; Martinez and Heymann, this volume, chapter 16) and the Centers for Disease Control have recently established a network of surveillance sites in the USA (Emerging Infections Programs—EIPS) (Berkelman, this volume, chapter 15). The establishment of a network of surveillance sites is an attractive approach to surveillance but there are a number of questions about the use of such sites that need to be answered. Surveillance sites are well suited to the monitoring of quantitative changes in prevalent infections, for example monitoring changes in antibiotic sensitivity patterns, but are they the most cost-effective way of detecting rare events such as the emergence of a new infection? Should surveillance sites be multipurpose or should they be built around groups with interest and expertise in a restricted area? How should the geographical position of surveillance sites be selected and how many are needed in a given area? Might strengthening of routine surveillance systems be a more cost-effective approach to disease surveillance than the establishment of focal surveillance sites, for the latter are often expensive to operate? Answers to some of these questions are likely to emerge during the next few years as more experience with surveillance sites accumulates.

Geographical information systems provide another approach to surveillance that may be very cost-effective. Environmental changes, for example changes in vegetation, can be monitored cheaply over extensive areas using satellite-derived information, and these changes may, in turn, be followed by changes in the incidence of infectious diseases. Earlier in this volume, the way in which satellite-derived data have been used to monitor changes in the epidemiology of malaria in Thailand (Gomes *et al*, this volume, chapter 7) and to monitor algal blooms and their possible relationship to outbreaks of cholera (Epstein, this volume, chapter 3) have been discussed. As more experience is gained in linking changes detected by global imaging with changes in disease patterns, geographical information systems are likely to play an increasingly important role in forecasting outbreaks, especially those of vector-borne diseases such as malaria.

Even when a surveillance system is working well it may be difficult to pick out from a mass of routine statistics the fact that something untoward is occurring. A simple way of doing this is to establish arbitrary rules that can be used to trigger an alert. This approach has been explored as a possible way of predicting epidemics of meningococcal meningitis in Africa. Based on experience in Burkina Faso, Moore and colleagues (1992) suggested that an outbreak of meningococcal meningitis is likely in the meningitis belt of Africa when the incidence rate reaches a figure of 15 cases or more per 100 000 population per week averaged over a period of two weeks in a population of around 50 000. In general, this prediction has worked reasonably well (Varaine *et al*, 1997), and a similar approach might be adopted for some other infectious diseases, such as cholera.

Diagnosis

An essential component of an effective surveillance system is an ability to make an accurate microbiological diagnosis. Surveillance may detect an increased incidence of unexplained fevers or of hepatitis in a given area, but the control measures that will be adopted will depend upon the nature of the microbiological diagnosis. Unfortunately, in many parts of the developing world, treatment of infectious diseases is undertaken on an empirical basis and microbiological diagnosis is either unavailable or not cost-effective. However, this does not apply to outbreak investigations in which accurate microbiological diagnosis is essential, even if this is expensive and difficult to achieve because the outbreak has occurred in a remote area. In such circumstances, new diagnostic tests which require little equipment may be especially helpful. For example, new dipstick assays for falciparum malaria, although too expensive for routine clinical use in many situations, may be extremely useful and cost-effective when used to investigate an outbreak of a severe febrile illness. A simple card test is available for the diagnosis of African trypanosomiasis and recently a skin biopsy test has been developed which can confirm a diagnosis of Ebola virus infection without the need for viral isolation (Rollin *et al*, this volume, chapter 8). Because of its extreme sensitivity and its ability to detect DNA in samples stored for a prolonged period under adverse environmental conditions, assays based on the polymerase chain reaction (PCR) have a tremendous potential for outbreak investigation, and this diagnostic approach is likely to be used increasingly frequently in the future. However, if reliance is to be placed on PCR diagnosis it is essential that effective quality control mechanisms are in place.

Response to an alert

The purpose of a surveillance system is to provide early warning of some unexpected event so as to allow a rapid and appropriate response. Determining what is an appropriate response in a particular situation can be very difficult. What should be done when a small cluster of cases of jaundice is reported in an African village or a report is received of two or three cases of bloody diarrhoea in a community in the UK? How much time and resources should be spent on investigating these outbreaks? What is the likelihood that major outbreaks of yellow fever or food poisoning are likely to occur? As surveillance systems expand, public health authorities are likely to be faced with situations such as these increasingly frequently. Ideally, responses should be based on a careful assessment of the likelihood of different outcomes, the costs of these outcomes and on the costs of possible responses (Foster, this volume, chapter 14; Roberts *et al*, this volume, chapter 13). For new infections, such as nvCJD, there may be no background epidemiological data to guide a decision as to what to do (Smith, this volume, chapter 10) However, for other infections there may be data from previous outbreaks that are helpful in determining the likely outcome of a particular series of events, and it is important that these databases should be expanded and made readily available to those faced with important public health decisions. Unfortunately, decisions on management of outbreaks are often based more on political and social considerations than on the results of careful scientific analysis of the situation (Palmer, this volume, chapter 11).

The nature of the response to an outbreak alert will depend upon the perceived magnitude of the threat. When this is high, a major response may be indicated, involving the participation of volunteers from outside the area of the outbreak and the involvement of international agencies. In such circumstances, co-operation between both national and international agencies is essential and examples of how this problem has been tackled during recent outbreaks are well described elsewhere in this volume (Moren, chapter 12).

Prevention

Tackling the major environmental and social factors that have contributed to the recent acceleration in the rate of appearance of new infections such as overpopulation, pollution, global warming and poverty is an enormous task and progress in these areas can be expected only over a prolonged period. However, some measures can be adopted now that are likely to have some benefit in the medium term. These include more rational use of antimicrobials and accelerated vaccine development.

Ways of reducing the inappropriate use of antibiotics need to be investigated both in industrialised and in developing countries so as to reduce unnecessary drug pressure on human pathogens. Possible approaches are a reduction in the use of antibiotics in animal husbandry, increasing controls over the prescription of specific antimicrobials by individual physicians and, in the developing world, reduction in the sale of antibiotics outside the official health care system. Even if pursued with vigour, such actions are likely to have only a limited impact on the development of drug resistance, and the development of new drugs will continue to be a priority. This raises particular problems for infections, such as malaria, that occur predominately in the third world. Pharmaceutical companies are reluctant to undertake the development of new drugs whose main market will be in poor countries and, even when they do, the cost of the new drug is likely to be high and thus beyond the means of the majority of people who need it most. Effective management of common infections of the third world such as malaria, pneumonia and dysentery is likely to become increasingly difficult in the near future.

The outlook in regard to vaccination is more promising. The past 20 years have seen great progress in the area of vaccinology, with the introduction into clinical use of polysaccharide/protein conjugate and recombinant vaccines and the development of DNA vaccines that are now in early clinical trials. Vaccine development offers at least an interim approach to the problem of some resurgent infections such as malaria and tuberculosis, and the development of an HIV vaccine, although extremely difficult, is not an impossibility. As vaccine technology advances, a situation may even be reached in which vaccines to new infections can be developed much more rapidly than at present, for example by use of the DNA approach. Development of vaccines against many of the major pathogens of the third world has been slow, in part for technical reasons but largely because of lack of resources. For example, the background knowledge needed to develop a conjugate vaccine that would provide long-lasting protection against group A meningococcal infection has been available for many years, yet development work in this area has only started recently, despite the fact that the group A meningococcus continues to cause havoc in Africa and elsewhere. Enhanced support for vaccine development probably offers the most promising medium-term approach to the control of several of the most important resurgent infections.

Conclusion

The end of the second millennium may represent the peak period for the emergence of new infections as some of the social and environmental changes that have characterized the twentieth century begin to slow down. During the 21st century, population growth is likely to stabilize, most arable land will have been exploited, most primary forests will have been cut down and an increasing proportion of the population will live in large urban centres of the type present in many parts of the developing world today. Global warming may facilitate the spread of some infectious diseases but is unlikely to have a major impact. However, the problem of antimicrobial resistance is likely to persist. The most promising approach to medium-term control of resurgent infections is likely to be through vaccination which may, in the not too far distant future, lead to eradication of some of the major infectious diseases prevalent today.

References

LeDuc JW. World Health Organisation strategy for emerging infectious diseases. *Journal of the American Medical Association*, 1996; **275**: 318–320

Moore PS, Plikaytis BD, Bolan GA *et al.* Detection of meningitis epidemics in Africa: a population-based analysis. *International Journal of Epidemiology*, 1992; **21**: 155–162

Varaine F, Caugan DA, Riou JY *et al.* Meningitis outbreaks and vaccination strategy. *Transactions of the Royal Society of Tropical Medicine and Hygiene*, 1997; **91**: 3–7

INDEX

Index compiled by A Campbell Purton

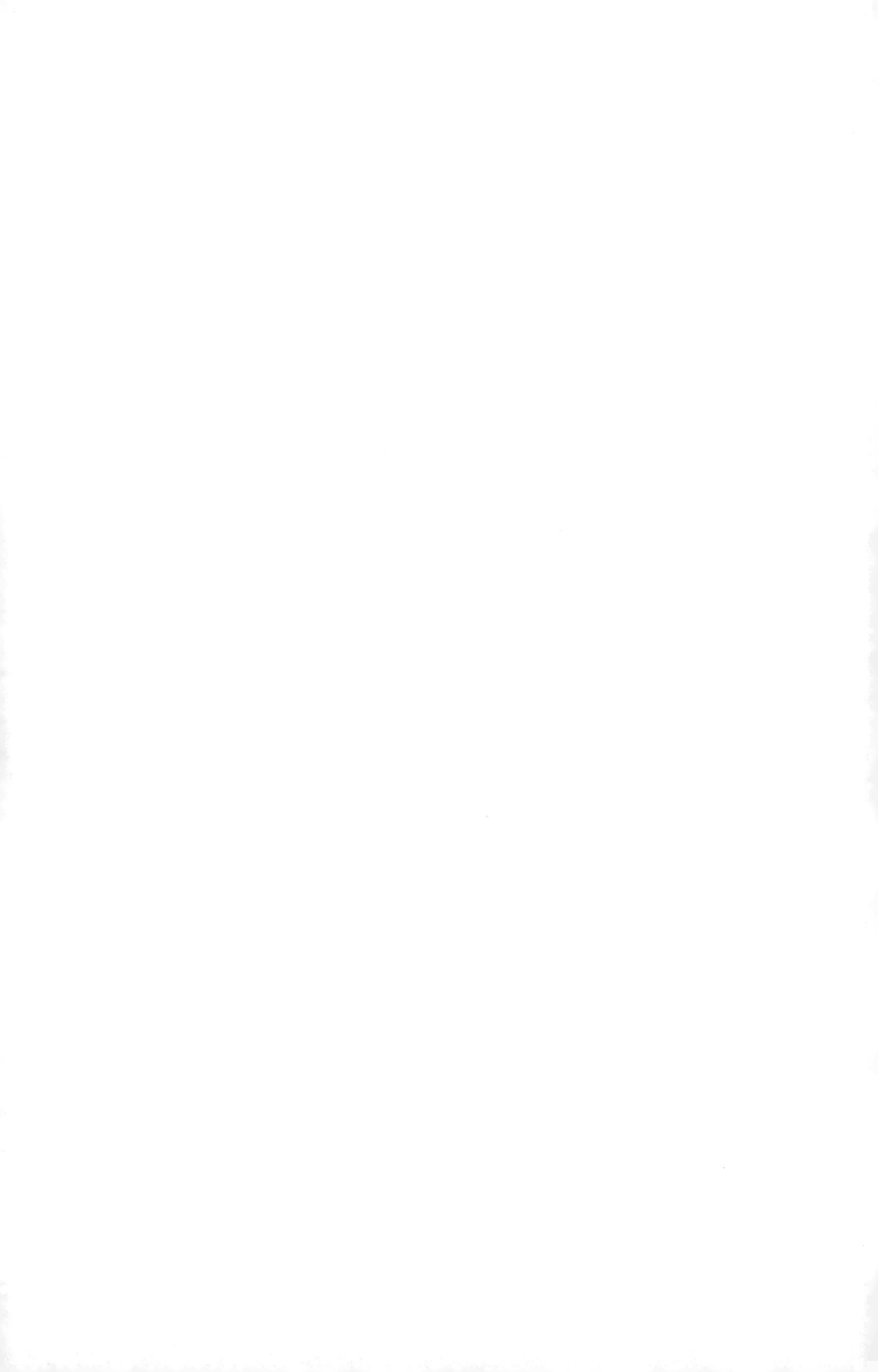